ENERGISTICS covers the objectives that we doctors strive for in our practices. If people understood these concepts, it would reduce much illness. ENERGISTICS includes exactly the concepts I have wanted our patients to understand.

> — *Alan S. Bensman, M.D., Psychiatrist, Medical Director, Minnesota Center of Health and Rehabilitation*

ENERGISTICS fills a needed function as a comprehensive guidebook for people who want to improve their physical, emotional and mental health. There is a wealth of information here, and a clear structure within which to use that information.

> — *David S. Bates, M.D.*

ENERGISTICS tells how to achieve an improved sense of well-being by paying attention to physical and mental aspects of the body's inner and outer environments. It avoids the traditional medical model of "curing disease" and instead tries to improve health. Practical information is presented step-by-step with enthusiasm, tempered by common sense.

> — *Michael Sananman, M.D.*

ENERGISTICS captures both the spirit and methods for vitalizing and empowering all levels of one's being. It is well-documented and researched and is supported by a sound philosophy. I highly recommend it to help make anyone's life greater.

> — *Lee Pulos, Ph.D.*

The very reading of ENERGISTICS will enhance your self-esteem ... to experience it is to feel affirmed. If everyone lived by the principles put forth here, we psychologists would ultimately be out of business. This is an excellent workbook for being the best one can be.

— *Cathy M. West, Ph.D.,*
Chief Clinical Psychologist, Youth
and Family Counseling Service

ENERGISTICS

Twelve Steps to Vitality, Health, and Well-Being

Phyllis Paullette

PaperJacks LTD.

TORONTO　NEW YORK

AN ORIGINAL

PaperJacks

ENERGISTICS

PaperJacks LTD

330 STEELCASE RD. E., MARKHAM, ONT. L3R 2M1
210 FIFTH AVE., NEW YORK, N.Y. 10010

PaperJacks edition published in April 1987

ISBN 0-7701-0568-8

Acknowledgments

I'm grateful to Nancy Parent of PaperJacks, Ltd., for encouraging me to write this book. I want to thank her and my editor, Jim Connor, for their trust and insight.

The following people made valuable contributions to this book by sharing professional knowledge, relating personal experiences, recommending books or lending from their personal libraries, reading the manuscript or simply helping me clarify my thoughts: Dorothy Ammon; Nancy Anderson; Wesley Balk, Ph.D.; Joy Bland; Dorothy Boen; James R. Boen, Ph.D.; Joie Bourisseau; Judy Boss; Judy Branson; Margot Breier; Philip Brunelle; David Buran, M.D.; Warren Burger, Ph.D.; Martha Burgess; William Castelli, M.D.; Claire Clay; Betty DeGuzman; David Dovenberg; George Montague Eberhardt; Erik Esselstyn, Ph.D.; J. Micki Esselstyn; Janet Harris Foord; John A. Foord; Judy Freedman; Joalta Danner Geidel; Wilma Gilkey; Linda Hoeschler; Janice Howard; Nancy Hubley; Penny Jacobs; Juanita Jacobson; Diana Wolfe Johnson;

Martha Keith; Barbara Krebs, Ph.D.; George Krebs, Ph.D.; Carolyn Z. Kostal; Loretta Lewis; Mary Longtine; Jeanne Morrisey; Roberta Perry; Alette Pontoppidan; Sue Poullette; Kathy Pratt, M.S., R.D.; John Prescott; Val Prescott; Asaf Qureshi, Ph.D.; Kilburg Reedy; Amy Simon; Howard Simon; Joseph Stokes III, M.D.; Kathleen C. Winn; and Rodger Winn, M.D.

There are others who shared wonderful experiences that for reasons of space could not fit into this book, and I thank them for their generosity. I also thank those whose personal accounts are included but who preferred to remain anonymous. (These individuals are identified in the text by pseudonymous first names.)

Special thanks to David S. Bates, M.D.; Alan S. Bensman, M.D.; Donna Gaffney, R.N., D.N.Sc.; Lee Pulos, Ph.D.; Michael Sananman, M.D.; Dr. Sidney B. Shane, M.D.; and Cathy M. West, Ph.D.

I'm especially grateful to Suzanne Morris and the Reverend Robert Corin Morris of Interweave Center for continued inspiration; the Berkeley Heights Public Library for special services; to Ann Buran for introducing me to Omega and the Musical Concoction; and to my friends all over the country for their gracious hospitality.

Hugs to Frank, Colin, and Michael for cheerfully suffering neglect through the writing process. A special round of applause to Colin, who met computer emergencies with calm expertise.

And finally, bouquets to my travel agent, Florence Parent, for her absolutely amazing connections.

To Ella and Phil, my mother and father

Contents

INTRODUCTION

What is Energistics?

Energistics is a twelve-step program designed to energize you to become all you can be. Each of the twelve steps represents an area in your life in which changes can be made to increase your energy potential. When you give attention to these twelve important areas, you may find:

- You have great zest for living.
- You are propelled and inspired by your creative mind, your healthy body, and your buoyant spirit.
- You love life with a passion.
- You are guided by your reason while you listen to your intuition.

- You welcome challenge as an opportunity to reach beyond the self.
- You trust a constant, never-ending inner source of strength and power.
- You feel wonderful.

How do you feel right now? Did you wake up this morning bursting with vitality? Is each day a new adventure? Are you filled with feelings of gratitude just for being alive?

Did you answer the preceding questions negatively? Is that why you picked up this book today? Did you wake up tired? Feeling low? Withered? Limited? Caffeine-dependent? Nicotine-dependent? Weighted down with worries or problems?

If so, you have a lot of company. Every day people who are stiff, short of breath, underexercised, oversized, and smokers are certified as "well" and "average" by medical doctors, but this doesn't mean that this kind of life is optimal for our species or that we must accept this reduced definition of living as our own.

We have all observed people whose energy seems abundant. They seem to have a glow that lights up the world around them. We tend to think of them as lucky, as exceptions, the products of good genes or — as special people who know secrets we don't share.

Genes do play a role in our available energy, but it's what we do with our genetic heritage that counts. Some people seem to be born on the run. Although their style appears energetic, it is often not a manifestation of true vitality but a sign of stress, obsession, neurosis, or addiction. I was once in awe of a neighbor who did everything fast, her cleaning and cooking were done before I was fully awake in the morning. I later learned that she was addicted to an amphetamine that was prescribed for her dog! Let's not be fooled by appearances.

Dramatic results can be attained when people give attention to the areas that have been neglected in their lives. Since we often get from life what we expect, I say, "Expect miracles!" At the same time, be realistic and remember that we are all mortal and operating within certain physical laws. While *Energistics* is not a recipe for the making of superwoman or superman, the results you gain from it may be super.

First, let's look at what could be causing you to feel different from those who seem to radiate energy:

- You may have forgotten how to eat, sleep, and play in ways that would renew and replenish you.
- You may have let inner entanglements like fear of failure, anger, or stress come between you and your energy source.
- You may have lost contact with your natural body.
- You may have become disconnected from yourself, people who are important to you, the essence of your work, or your social groups.

These are habits, and habits can be changed. People *can* grow in chosen directions. There's always room for new growth, and it's our nature to want to grow better instead of just older. Because there's always another moun-

tain to climb, coming to terms with our genetic requirements, habits, emotional and environmental influences
can be a lifelong task. The *Energistics* twelve-point system
is designed to facilitate this process.

No doubt everyone has experienced a feeling of bound-
less energy at least once. Remember the day you got your
first car? The first time you fell in love? The game that
your team won — because of you? You glowed. You
sparkled. You were so energized you seemed to defy gravity. Your energy was almost visible!

Have you thought about how to recapture this wonderful feeling? Or does it seem out of reach, an impossible
dream? The source of this energy is still ours. In the absence
of serious health problems, it's possible to recapture this
wonderful, weightless vitality.

Energy is all around us and within us. It nourishes
us, contains us, perhaps even *is* us. The planet we live
on is one interrelated system, and energy may be what
connects us to it, to life, and to one another. *Energistics*
can help you strengthen these connections.

The energists I interviewed for this book shared
hundreds of suggestions for raising energy, among them
ways to:

- Let go of fatigue and negativity by conquering
  energy-draining habits and obstacles.
- Encourage natural body wisdom through
  increased self-awareness.
- Take control of your life and stop trying to control the lives of others.
- Deal with stress productively and make decisions
  that don't conflict with biological needs.

- Cooperate with yourself to become more alive, more vigorous, more energetic.
- Stop fracturing yourself into parts and rejoin your body, mind and spirit into the one great person that is you.

You can do a great deal for yourself. While many good programs exist that require someone else to perform a service for you, they are outside the realm of this book, which concentrates upon you and what you can do for yourself.

I am not a medical person and this book is not a substitute for medical advice. I assume that if you have a problem that requires professional help, you will seek it. Doctors and hospitals are important and we cannot do without them, but there are many levels of health beyond the absence of physical illness. In this non-medical realm your feelings of well-being may be more dependent upon the daily choices you make, rather than those your doctors make for you. If you want to be *really* well, what I call *vitally alive*, you must be actively involved, making conscious and informed daily choices about your well-being.

My interest is in helping healthy people become healthier, more energetic, and more alive. When I use the word *energy* in this book, I am using the colloquial, not the scientific meaning, to define a quality of consciousness, an attitude and a feeling of extreme well-being. I do not recognize "bad energy," only well-directed or not well-directed energy. When you say you're "feeling good" or "not feeling good" (aside from specific discomfort arising from the presence of disease), you may be referring to your energy state. When your energy feels good, it's flowing, well directed, working for you. When it doesn't, it's blocked or stuck. Getting unstuck is what this book is about.

What You Love Grows

We know that what we resist persists. What we ignore continues to plague us and get in our way. Whatever we exclude from our awareness expands in negative ways. Unweeded gardens, unanswered phone calls, lost buttons, unbalanced checkbooks and untended relationships, along with life's other little details, have a way of mushrooming into seemingly insurmountable entanglements. These eventually become energy blocks.

An important underlying principle of the *Energistics* system is summed up in the short phrase: What you love grows. The energy you focus in any direction expands this area into greater importance in your life. Everything you choose to love (or give your attention to) becomes you, just as your food becomes you. This includes your friends, leisure activities, vocational commitments, and the environment in which you have surrounded yourself. All can be great energizers.

Obviously, it isn't possible in the space of a day to give active attention to everything. Choosing to take conscious and deliberate control of where to direct your attention is what I call "love." Here's an example: If you love playing the drums, becoming a good drummer will be effortless. You don't have to sweat and suffer over it because you love to practice. Doing it is its own reward, so you keep at it. "I am a drummer," you hear yourself say. Into your life come people with similar talents and interests — a guitar player, a vocalist, a sound technician. Eventually, there will be a club in which to perform. You have now traveled from interest to identity to social contacts to environment, maybe even to a new avocation or vocation, all of which started with your love of drumming. Drumming will be a source of energy as well as relaxation.

If you love tennis, the same thing happens. You will play tennis, you will attract friends who play tennis, watch tennis on TV, and perhaps read books on "inner" as well as "outer" tennis. Soon you may be terrific at tennis. Playing tennis will become energizing exercise.

What we love and give our attention to grows in direct proportion to how much we love it. Choosing well and following these interests passionately have the potential to change and revitalize us. The corollary to this is that whatever in our lives needs growth or improvement needs first to be loved.

Perhaps you are wondering how you can love something nebulous and intangible like your energy source. With this book as your guide, make a commitment to give this subject your active attention for the period of time you need to enhance your available energy. Make a decision to make yourself and your energy your number-one priority for this period. Mark your projected scheduling of each step on your calendar now and be realistic enough to allow for unforeseen events. You may see results sooner than you expect.

Writing notes to yourself and doing the written exercises as you read will speed your progress. It is my hope that

Energistics will stretch you, stimulate you, and bring your own hidden knowledge into your awareness where you can act upon it to create a more vital self.

The overriding connection that we have to our inner selves, to one another, and to our world is our energy. This is what makes us like nature and unlike even our most advanced machines. We are incredibly well designed. We are magnificent.

Getting Started

In the years I struggled with ups and downs in my own available energy and in the two years I spent interviewing and researching in preparation for writing this book, I found there is not one simple answer — there is no one diet or regimen that will cause everyone to burst with vitality. Because each of us is unique, our energy needs at any given time are diverse. What works for one of us today may not work for another person until later.

This is why there is no single approach in this book, no one magic potion for lighting the fire inside yourself, but many energy-expanding ideas from diverse sources. *Energistics* contains ideas from health experts, common-sense backed up by new research, accounts of other people's personal energy-transforming experiences, and my own practical, do-it-yourself suggestions in twelve areas. Like intersecting circles comprising a whole sphere, the twelve steps in the *Energistics* program are:

1. Invigorating Physical Exercise

Energistics focuses on you and what you can discover about your own needs. We know that when we do everything the same as we always have, our life is likely to remain the same. When significant improvements are sought, change is part of the process. This book is arranged in a way to most easily facilitate change, so do begin at the beginning and proceed in the order given. Because some changes are easier to make than others, the easier ones are presented before those that are more difficult and subjects close at hand before those further from your control. Furthermore, practicing the exercises in one chapter will make it easier to accomplish the skills presented in the next. For example, I believe that learning to breathe more efficiently is easier than becoming an athlete if you have always led a sedentary life. However, once you are breathing better and taking in more oxygen, you may feel more vigorous, so getting yourself to the gym for regular exercise will be easier and more enjoyable. This is why you will find breathing presented before physical exercise. And since engaging in physical exercise encourages better sleep, exercise is presented before sleep, and so forth.

On occasion, however, there may be good reasons to break this order. If you are exhausted because you can't sleep, getting a good night's sleep will be your top priority. If you know that fear and worry are keeping you awake, you should skip from the Sleep section to the Fears section, especially The Worry Quiz. It's no use reading about love or nutrition or the energizing effects of visualization until you get a good night's sleep!

You can do energy work from the outside in or from the inside out, so both approaches are included. Since the outside or physical part of ourselves is generally more accessible to us and more readily changed, we'll start with the physical: well-nourished, refreshed, and active people have more fun, more awareness, more energy, more *life*. In Part II we'll switch directions and discuss how inner states have much to do with our physical health and available energy.

PART I

A VITALLY ALIVE PHYSICAL SELF

Step 1. Invigorating Physical Exercise: The #1 Vitamin

If you could take a safe and proven pill that would give you more energy, help you maintain your ideal size, lower your blood pressure, make you appear more vital and attractive, let you have a good night's sleep, add years to your life, and give you a terrific mood lift, you'd take it, right? You wouldn't even think twice about it.

There is such a pill. It's called *exercise*. Some people call it "the #1 vitamin" because it makes everything else work better. Because it gives you a mood lift, and induces a feeling of well being, exercise is the best and quickest way to raise your energy level. The following are other reasons to exercise. If you already practice a complete and balanced exercise program, you can marvel at all your routine is doing for you:

- Exercise can help you become a smaller size, even at the same weight, by firming up your muscles.

- Exercise makes you burn calories. Instead of ruining your health and sapping your energy with nutrient-restricting reducing diets, exercise longer and on a regular basis. A well-conditioned person consumes calories at a faster rate during waking hours even when not exercising! Exercise also reduces the appetite and makes the metabolism more efficient. It gives your skin a glow and your step a lilt that sedentary people don't have. When you exercise regularly, you stand straighter, which makes you look better regardless of your weight.

- People who exercise regularly report that they are more effective on *and* off the job. Nowadays, exercise has become the mark of the high achiever. In a Gallup Poll, 62% of people who exercise reported feeling more energy throughout the day than they had prior to exercising. A full 45% of those polled agreed with the statement: "Fitness brings a better love life."[1]

- Running, one of the most popular ways to exercise, has been shown to combat moderate depression.[2] This may be because it is an aerobic exercise and therefore stimulates the production of endorphins. Endorphins (the body's natural opiates) are what bring on the good feelings called the "runner's high." Running also encourages creativity; runners often claim that their running session is when they think, when their best ideas appear.

- Exercise counters stress, balances your energy, and increases your alertness, allowing you to experience your optimal self.
- Exercise can lower blood pressure and total serum cholesterol while increasing the levels of the protective cholesterol carrier H.D.L.[3] (More on this later.)
- Exercise helps the heart pump more blood with less effort and allows it to rest longer between beats. It also increases the ability of the muscles to extract and use the oxygen the blood delivers.
- Exercise may help people avoid osteoporosis, diabetes, and strokes.[4]
- Exercise can retard, even reverse, the aging process. Not only do you get a boost of energy today, but by exercising now, you have a greater chance of having a vigorous old age. It's like putting money in the "energy bank."
- Even moderate exercise can extend your life. Moderate means walking three miles a day or systematically climbing stairs or engaging in sports to the extent of using 2,000 calories or more a week.

A 1984 study of almost seventeen thousand middle-aged and older alumni of Harvard University provided the first strong scientific evidence that people who are active live longer. The results are clear: People who exercise have strong cardiovascular systems, while sedentary people have more cardiovascular disease. Dr. Bruce Dan, editor of the sports issue of *The Journal of the American Medical Association*, commented upon the report: "We can now prove that large numbers of Americans are dying from sitting on their behinds."[5]

My grandfather didn't spend much time on his behind. I made a home movie of him hoeing his patch of sweet corn when he was ninety-seven, and a video of his one hundredth birthday party. He presided over the proceedings magnanimously and the same day screened the video for his younger and less-mobile friends in a nursing home. His secret? He expressed the importance of a strong religious belief and "keeping my legs moving." He was walking when he died.

A follow-up to the Harvard study considered not only cardiovascular fitness but deaths from all causes.[6] It confirmed what my grandfather knew intuitively: Exercise helps people live longer and have less disease.[7] While scientists seek to determine why this is true, walk, run, swim, and pedal as though your life depends upon it. It probably does.

More Oxygen, More Energy

One reason exercise makes us feel so good is that it improves our intake of oxygen. Breathing is more than a ventilation system for the body. Breathing is the way we carry oxygen, our primary nutrient, our "handle" to our emotions, and is basic to our well-being. What we in the Western world overlook is that breathing is an exercise anyone can do. It is not necessary to be in motion to practice breathing, yet it is the most neglected physical exercise in the Western world.

As you are reading this book you are consuming about

sixteen quarts of air a minute, and three times this if you go for a run.[8] When breathing is so easy and automatic, why should we unless we happen to be opera singers or bassoon players bother to think about it? What's in it for us?

How we breathe can energize or depress us. A close relationship exists between the breath, the autonomic nervous system, and emotional states. This relationship has been largely neglected by Western medicine, but has been researched thoroughly in yoga science for thousands of years.

You may have heard or read about advanced yogis who can perform phenomenal feats (stopping the heart voluntarily or deliberately altering their body temperature, for example). These acts aren't feats of magic, but involve real bodily control, based upon altered states made possible by the understanding of the subtle role the breath plays in regulating the body. The reason the yogis demonstrate these feats (it takes great effort on their part) is to prove to us that much more physical control is possible than we in the Western hemisphere ordinarily realize.

We don't have to go to the extremes the yogis do to obtain health benefits. Understanding a few simple facts about breathing can be of practical use and may make an appreciable and immediate difference in one's feeling of well-being.

The exhalation (out-breath) is the calming part of the breath cycle, and the inhalation (in-breath) the energizing part. The inhalation energizes because of its connection with the sympathetic nervous system, the portion of the nervous system that becomes more active during emergencies or stress.

The advantage of understanding and manipulating the breathing mechanism is most apparent during strenuous exercise or athletic competition. The finest athletes may be those who have learned to coordinate their breathing with the requirements of their sport, but the rest of us can benefit from simply becoming more conscious of our breathing during any type of intense activity. Breathing out explosively while hitting a volleyball may give the blow more power. While preparing to pack a strong punch into your tennis backhand, you might breathe out or breathe into a word like "wow!" The simultaneous expiration of the breath will give your stroke more power in the same way that shouting "Kiai!" does while executing a karate maneuver. Whether the effect is psychological or physical or both, it works.

While aerobic dancing, a skilled breather can deliberately slow breathing to reduce the pulse rate, resulting in more endurance and a greater level of safety. If you are a runner, you can extend your endurance by paying attention to your breathing and coordinating it with your strides. Use an uneven count, longer on the exhalation, coordinated with your steps. For example, using a 4-step exhalation and a 3-step inhalation (or a 5:4 or a 3:2) can generate extra endurance on a long run. Experiment to see what works for you. Long, even, and natural breaths are best for skiing, so don't allow fear to cause you to hold your breath. Holding your breath while skiing invites disaster.

You may have noticed that emitting a sigh (a long out-breath) calms you. An involuntary gasp (a fast in-breath) activates the "fight or flight" response and makes you ready for action. These actions don't have to be involuntary, but can be controlled. The advice "Take a deep breath" before taking angry or stressful action is contrary to our physiology; it focuses on the inhalation, which activates the sympathetic nervous system. Just what you don't need when you are trying to relax! So the results are exactly the opposite of what is intended. Instead, when you feel a sudden burst of anger coming on, stop and exhale a long, slow breath. Repeat, and let yourself relax before you take action.

We can use breathing techniques to relax, to pep ourselves up, to feel energized, to calm our heartbeat during vigorous exercise, or to go to sleep. We can breathe in a way that cleans bad air from our lungs. Control over our breathing gives us increased control over ourselves and may be used to help regulate emotions.

The "Ins" and "Outs" of Breathing

Becoming a more sophisticated breather is not difficult. Here are some breath exercises to try:

Baby Breathing   If you have access to a newborn baby, watch the baby, then imitate his breathing; babies do it perfectly.

Yawning Well   Observe and imitate your own yawn. When you yawn, you relax, engage the diaphragm, completely fill your lungs, then expell fully, all of which are good features to incorporate into your habitual breathing patterns. Breathing with your yawning skills can give you more oxygen.

The Dictionary Method of Breathing   Lie on the floor and put a heavy book, like a dictionary or a telephone book, over your diaphragm, which is located just above your naval. Practice bouncing it up and down. This helps you find the place from which you want to breathe.

Diaphragmatic Breathing   Lie on your back and place your right hand on your diaphragm (just above your navel) and your left hand in the middle of your chest. As you breathe, try to feel the right hand moving up and down freely with the breath. Try to keep the left hand still. It should not be moving at all. When you feel a great difference between one hand and the other, you are breathing correctly.

Beware of tight clothing. Breathing in a shallow way is often the result of years of wearing tight and constricting clothing. It can result in diminished energy and can interfere with your ability to register and experience a full range of emotions.

Relaxing Breathing   Observe your normal breathing and count ("One thousand one, one thousand two ..."), marking the length of each breath segment. How many counts does it take for you to breathe in and how many for you to breathe out? Four? Five? Try making each inhalation and each exhalation equal in length. Connect each inhalation and exhalation so that there are no stops or gasps, just a smooth breath in and a smooth breath out. *Do not hold your breath!* Always tell yourself to put your breathing back on "automatic" — normal and easy — before you end the session.

2:1 Breathing   Once you have mastered relaxing breathing, try to make the exhalation *twice* as long as the inhalation. This is very relaxing and can temporarily reduce pulse rates and lower blood pressure. *Caution: This is not a substitute for medical intervention.*

Breathing And Sex   Some women have learned to have orgasms for the first time simply by learning to keep breathing, rather than holding the breath when feeling intense emotion. One woman told me she can control when to have her orgasms by elongating the exhalation like 2:1 breathing and by visualizing herself "dropping down" into the orgasm when she chooses. Before the breathing training, her habit was to hold her breath whenever she felt intense emotion. (Holding the breath or breathing erratically can cut off physical sensation.) Now both the breathing and the visualization relax her sufficiently to make it possible to have simultaneous orgasms with her partner.

Breathing for the Long Term   One very important reason to learn efficient breathing is to prepare for your vigorous and energetic old age. Studies show that a lot of what is thought to be symptoms of aging is the result of a diminished intake of oxygen. Dr. Marcus Bach writes, "Effective breathing among Americans drops from one hundred percent at birth to sixty percent in middle age to forty percent of capacity at age seventy-five. All other functions, such as nerve conduction, metabolism, and cardiac output, deteriorate in relation to a drop in breathing efficiency."[9]

Proper exercise can restore this oxygen-carrying facility by as much as 40%, according to *The Journal of the American Medical Association*.[10] With aerobic exercise the heart can actually increase its capacity for pumping oxygen through your body, but the rest of the body also benefits from increased oxygen. Exercised muscles use oxygen more efficiently, which maintains their endurance. Disuse leads to muscle deterioration. "Use it or lose it" is wise advice.

Since oxygen is what keeps us alert and youthful, habitual deep and efficient breathing is the way to best use it. More oxygen over the course of a lifetime means more energy, so exercise your breathing mechanism and feel wonderful.

Aerobic Exercise

You want your exercise to be efficient, right? You don't have time to spend half the day at the gym? Aerobic exercises will give you the greatest improvement for the time spent than any other physical exercise. Aerobic means "with oxygen" and refers to exercise that increases the oxygen use. Aerobic exercise keeps your pulse elevated to 70% to 80% of maximum capacity for a minimum of twelve minutes of steady nonstop exercise. Walking, running, bicycling, jumping rope, cross-country skiing, rowing, and aerobic dancing are aerobic. Golf, weight lifting, tennis, and hatha yoga are not aerobic.

In order to build better fitness, it's necessary to push yourself a little beyond what you normally do. Doing only what is easy will maintain the current fitness level. Going beyond or overloading builds for tomorrow.[11]

To compare your rate of exertion with your optimal training level, learn to find your pulse, either on your wrist or at the large artery in your neck. Watch a clock or wristwatch with a second hand and count the number of beats you feel within six seconds. Multiply this number by ten for your heartbeats per minute. Learn to take your pulse both while resting and while exercising, and make allowances for being between beats when the six seconds are up by adding a five. If your number is between nine and ten beats, your heartbeats per minute become ninety-five.

There are several ways to calculate your optimal degree of exertion. In his book, *Fit or Fat?*, trainer Covert Bailey suggests that you first find your resting heart rate by taking your pulse several times during the day and averaging it. Write your average resting heart rate here: _____

Bailey gives this formula for learning your maximum heart rate: 220 Minus Your Age = Your Maximal Heart Rate. *Do not exercise at this maximal heart rate!* Use it in only in your calculations. Write your maximal heart rate here: _____

To determine your training heart rate, Bailey proposes this formula: Maximum Heart Rate minus Resting Heart Rate × 65% plus resting Heart Rate = Training Heart Rate (or Target Zone.) Write your training heart rate here: _____

Bailey's example: A forty-year-old has a resting heart rate of 70. To calculate her training heart rate: 180 - 70 × 65% + 70 = 141.5. When this person exercises, the proper heart rate to maintain is 141-142 beats per minute.[12]

If you are over thirty-five and haven't been exercising or have a history of heart problems, forget the preceding information and go to your doctor for a stress electro-cardiogram. This is an expensive test, so you may be invited to take a less costly test, the resting electrocardiogram. Covert Bailey suggests that this test will tell you only how safe it is to rest, which is not really what you want to know.[13] So press for the active test, the one that monitors you while you are exercising. Then you will have the confidence to work out with gusto.

Working below your optimal training heart rate maintains but doesn't build fitness. Working above is dangerous and counterproductive. When you become more experienced, you can control your heartbeat and the amount of exertion by speeding up or slowing down your pace and intensity of exercise and controlling your breathing. Know yourself and respect your capacity.

Wear loose-fitting, well ventilated clothing and drink plenty of fluids before, during, and after your workout.

Your Other Exercise Routine

Aerobic exercise, as described in the last section, is only half of your exercise program. You need two kinds of exercise to stay fit: one that speeds you up and gets you moving, and one that slows you down and encourages relaxation. Hatha yoga fills the bill exactly for the latter. Hatha also encourages body awareness and important joint and muscle flexibility. When you design a balanced exercise program for yourself, you will include both aerobic and relaxing exercise or some variation of both, respecting your needs and capabilities.

If you seek more emphasis on building strength and sinewy muscles, add weight training, regular work with a rowing machine, or use other specially designed exercises for this purpose. But don't neglect aerobics and flexibility training. These are basic to an increased sense of well-being and the likelihood of a long and healthy life, so they should be your primary considerations.

When you design your own program, decide what your own body needs and be aware of the benefits and limitations of the activities you have chosen.

Hatha yoga is a practical system of exercise that expands physical and mental self-awareness and calms the mind as it develops a strong and flexible body. This centuries-old tradition leads systematically from physical exercises to breathing skills to better concentration and beyond.[14]

Hatha yoga consists of stretches and stationary postures that work one muscle against another naturally and — when performed under the guidance of a good teacher — more efficiently and with greater safety than a weight machine. The different postures are held for several seconds or minutes, then alternated with periods of rest and relaxation. Aside from the good physical exercise, this practice helps one gain control of the tension-relaxation response. When you are practiced at tension — how to create it, how to let it go — it becomes easier to deal with life's unavoidable stresses.

The goals of hatha yoga — physical well-being, increased self-awareness, balance, harmony, inner peace — lead to a greater capacity for concentration. A regular hatha practice teaches you to sense your body's moods and pulses. Becoming aware of these subtle body energies is an effective way for reconnecting the body and the mind, a balance that is basic to vibrant good health. Through the quiet that comes with hatha and meditation, you can learn to recognize which parts of yourself have been neglected and need attention and how to strengthen them. In addition, knowing your body well helps you to be aware of small changes. This awareness can act as an early warning system, alerting you to signs before they become symptoms, signs perhaps more subtle than your physician can detect in a physical examination.

Doing a daily hatha practice and an aerobic activity ensures that whatever physical mobility, flexibility, endurance, cardiovascular fitness, or strength you have today you will still have tomorrow. These benefits go far beyond what is offered by any single exercise or sport.

Before doing the more strenuous activities, always warm up slowly with hatha yoga or other gentle stretches. (Don't bounce when you stretch. Just assume the posture, hold, and slowly let go.) Cool down after hard exertion, continuing the same exercise at a slower pace. If you wish, finish with more stretching to avoid stiffness.

Hatha yoga traditions vary — from very gentle stretching to very vigorous acrobatics. All hatha includes increased breath awareness and oxygen intake that allow some degree of "turning the clock back." Many hatha devotees find themselves walking and moving as they did when they were younger.

I do not provide detailed instructions for hatha yoga postures here because it's a complex system, and I believe that it's important for you to work with a teacher. Find one who is well qualified and who will look out for your health and safety.

I think hatha yoga is wonderful. If, however, you feel it's weird or foreign, don't deprive yourself of the stretches hatha offers. The book *Stretching*, by Bob Anderson

(Random House, 1980), shows you how to get the benefits of the same stretches within an exercise-program context.

There are so many ways to exercise. The following will benefit your heart and increase your use of oxygen: aerobic workout, jogging, fast walking, bicycling, jumping rope, cross-country skiing, swimming, and skating.

Other activities, such as Eastern martial arts like judo, karate, and *t'ai chi*, offer good discipline and physical training, but, like hatha, may not include aerobic exercise.

Rebounding — jumping on a mini-trampoline — can be temporarily energizing and is fun to do, but is not demanding enough to really keep a person fit. It can be a "starter exercise" after illness or be of some use to those who are very overweight. Healthy and hardy people need more. Certain kinds of dancing can provide a complete exercise program if designed properly and performed regularly. Imaginative new ways to enjoy exercise seem to appear weekly. There are aerobic tap dancing, Jazzercise, aerobic yoga, and many more. Square dancing is great for older people. Surely there's a perfect exercise routine for you.

Evaluating Your Exercise Program — Quiz

1. Does your exercise program include aerobic activity that raises your pulse into your target zone?
2. Does this elevated pulse level continue for 20 minutes or more?
3. Do you do this three times a week or more?
4. Do you find that you breathe hard, but can still talk?

5. Do you warm up before exercising and cool down afterward and include some stretching?

6. Do you cool down after a vigorous workout so that your pulse rate drops to under 120 beats per minute before you resume normal activities?

7. Does your program also include a routine for flexibility that challenges you to stretch to your maximum comfortable stretching level three times a week or more?

8. Does your program include upper and lower body work as well as left- and right-side exercise?

9. Does your program include some work on muscular endurance?

10. Do you enjoy your exercise sessions, look forward to them, and leave feeling more relaxed than when you started?

Give yourself 2 points for every yes, 1 point for every "most of the time," and 0 points for a negative answer. Eighteen points and above: you must be a perfect "10"; 13-18 points: you're in good shape; 3-13 points: reevaluate your exercise program using previous suggestions; below 2 points: you are not a plant! Start moving.

Too Much of a Good Thing — Quiz

Exercise is terrific, but beyond a certain point, more is not necessarily better. If you suspect that your exercise program is taking over your life, or if you scored a perfect

20 on the previous quiz, think about whether this area of your life is in balance.

Too much exercise can make you tired and haggard as easily as can undereating; either way, you may be losing muscle instead of fat. Switching exercise every other day is a good way to let your muscles repair: For example, jog or do an aerobic workout on Monday, Wednesday, and Friday, and hatha yoga or stretching exercises on Tuesday, Thursday, and Saturday.

Check any of the following that apply to you:

1. Your knees (or back, ankles, feet) hurt.
2. You have to do more and more in order to feel good.
3. Your exercising has become more important than the people in your life.
4. Your periods have stopped (for women).
5. You are nervous and depressed in spite of your continued vigorous exercise program.
6. You are tired all the time.
7. You cannot relax except after your exercise.
8. You have lost weight unexpectedly.
9. You have a cold a lot of the time.
10. Is your exercising program beginning to feel like an obsession? Or maybe it just isn't fun anymore.

A "yes" to 2 or more of these questions could indicate that you are overexercising. Stop for a few days and see what happens. If the symptons disappear, reevaluate your program. Is it balanced? Moderate? Do you do vigorous work every other day to give your muscles time to heal between sessions? There may be other reasons for these symptoms. Slow down. Listen to your body. Check it out.

If you are a runner and answered "yes" to numbers, 3, 7, and/or 10, you may want to stop running and substitute another rigorous activity like swimming or biking for a few weeks in order to evaluate the role that running plays in your life.

Research done by Dr. Connie Chan found that runners, when prevented from running, were "more depressed, anxious, tense, and confused than active runners."[15] Running has its psychological benefits, but those who can cope with life only by running, who need running in order not to be depressed, who have no other way of dealing with stress, are "jogging-dependent," according to Dr. Chan. If you find that you fit this description, stop temporarily and try to find other activities that elevate your moods and restore you equilibrium. Should you ever be prevented from running, you will have something equally satisfying upon which to fall back.

Exercise Alibis

You never exercise? Afraid to start?

The reason given most often by non-exercisers is "not enough time." This is a weak reason, since exercise makes the rest of the day more efficient, causes people to sleep better (sometimes for a shorter length of time), and gives the exerciser more pep. Putting exercise sessions on your calendar is the only way to find time on a regular basis. Once the routine is established, the time in which to do it will create itself.

A reason given less often, but a real obstacle for many, is fear — of commitment, of change, of embarrassment, of getting hurt.

People can get hurt exercising. But getting no exercise at all is a sure way to harm yourself. Muscle deterioration from being sedentary goes on silently and painlessly — until you discover backaches or other problems that develop from flaccid muscles that no longer can support your bones. During sedentary periods, fat can replace muscle without your being aware of it.

When you look over the benefits that exercise bestows on your blood pressure, your cardiovascular system, your joints and muscles, your overall health and longevity, you have to conclude that the sedentary life is by far the more dangerous.

When designing your exercise program, remember that you need one routine to slow and relax you and one routine to raise your pulse into your target zone.

Aerobic activities: _____

_____

_____

How often?: _____

_____

_____

How long?: _____

_____

_____

Relaxing stretching activities: _____

_____

How often?: _____

_____

How long?: _____

_____

Translate this program into hours in your day and insert these into your calendar on appropriate days for the next few months. Let exercise become your habit, knowing that your habits "become" you.

Step 2.   Revitalizing Sleep

You can't soar with the eagles in the morning if
you hoot with the owls the night before.
— Folk Wisdom

Some people can't get to sleep at night. Others fall asleep
easily but need so much sleep that it interferes with their
lives. Some people fall asleep in the middle of the day,
but not at night. Others can fall asleep at bedtime, but
awaken to spend the middle of the night sleepless and
the next day dragging themselves around in a state of
fatigue. Some people think they are not sleeping when
they are. Others are too anxious to sleep — sometimes
because they're worrying that they cannot get to sleep!
Sleep itself (and why we need it) is something of a
mystery. Sleep researchers are finding that not everyone

needs the standard eight hours.[16] Although the average seems to be about seven and a half, three hours in either direction is considered normal. Some adults need five, others ten. And some can function well on less than five. We're all different. A good night's sleep for you may be all wrong for someone else.

The ABZzzz's of Insomnia

A good day is preceded by a good night, but the reverse is also true. What you do during the day has a lot to do with how well you sleep at night. It is not known whether a quiet and passive daytime life-style is the cause or result of insomnia, but one way to cope with it is to be more active during the day.

Researchers have found that insomniacs spend more time watching television, shopping, and relaxing than good sleepers. Their daytime thoughts were different from those of good sleepers.[17] Insomniacs tended to think about their physical environment, various forms of passive relaxations, like planning their TV-watching schedule or thinking about a book they had read or what was on the news. Good sleepers spent their time thinking about interpersonal relationships and their families.

If you are active and energetic, you get tired at night and go to sleep more easily. Daily exercise is the best way to enhance sound sleep. If you aren't sleeping well and you aren't part of the majority of people who exercise regularly, this is the obvious first step.

You do exercise? If you are still troubled by insomnia,

here are additional steps you can take to get a better night's sleep.

A Sleep/Energy Log   You can learn a lot about your sleep habits by keeping track of how well you slept, how you felt the next day, what you had for supper, whether you drank alcohol, what your daytime activity level was on the days that you slept better or worse. You might include what you were thinking about while you were not sleeping.

Keep Yourself on Schedule   The best daytime alertness occurs on a stable schedule of eating and sleeping. If you need to go to bed later than usual, do so, but always rise at the same time. Sleeping late on the weekend can confuse the message and, subsequently, the sleep schedule. And, unless you are a good sleeper, don't nap. Save up your sleeping for nighttime. If you go to bed only when you are tired, you are more likely to be able to go to sleep.

Worry Notes   Keep a note pad by your bed and write down everything that's on your mind before you go to sleep. Include any unfinished business of the past day and any reminders for the next day. Entries as mundane as "Don't forget the dry cleaning" can clear your mind and allow for more restful sleep. If habitual worry about decisions or life events is keeping you awake, see Step 11. Sometimes just worrying about the fact that you are not sleeping keeps you awake. Write that down as well.

Eat Lightly   Digesting a heavy meal may be distracting you from a good night's sleep. The old advice "Eat like a king in the morning, a prince at noon, and a pauper at night" is good for sleep problems. If you must eat before bedtime, choose "sleepy" food; low-protein food (fruits, vegetables and whole grains) is easiest to digest. One type of protein that seems to encourage sleep is L-tryptophan, found in turkey and milk. Warm the milk before bedtime and sleep like a baby.

Love Your Bedroom   Decorate your bedroom so that it is restful and pleasing to your eye. (See Step 4). Give attention to the linens and pillow and the quality of the mattress. Notice the placement of the windows. (Does a streetlight keep you awake or the sun wake you too early? Blackout shades are the answer here.) See that the lighting is pleasant and near the bed so that you can read for a few moments before dozing off. Wear ear plugs if the room is situated close to unavoidable outside noise. Most people sleep better when they do not see the face of a clock. Check the temperature and humidity. Give your bedroom your loving attention. After all, you spend one third of your life there.

Isolate Your Bedroom from Your Life   If possible, devote the bedroom to sleeping. Leave work in another room (in a one-room apartment, leave it behind a screen in another part of the room). Bring into your bedroom only those things that make you feel good, that do not suggest conflicts.

Your Sleep Wardrobe   Give some attention to the clothes you sleep in, if any. Some people sleep best in the nude. Others prefer to wear soft, flannellike fabrics. Decide what is best for you.

Yoga or Relaxation   Doing slow and gentle yoga (not vigorous exercise) or a structured relaxation routine before bedtime can induce drowsiness. (See Steps 1 and 5.)

Your Bedtime Ritual   Develop a ritual that you do

every night in the same order. Check the locks, put out the cat, lay out tomorrow's clothes, floss your teeth, whatever. Be consistent. For most people, a hot bath before bedtime is sleep-inducing and is a good way to let your body slow down. (For some, a hot bath is energizing. See what works for you.) Your regular bedtime habits alert your body that sleep time is coming and give it the message to adjust to the sleep mode.

Evaluate Addictions   Smokers don't sleep as well as non-smokers, researchers tell us.[18] Stimulants, even prescription drugs, can induce sleeplessness. Check with your doctor or pharmacist.

Beware of Caffeine   If you want to use caffeine-containing products, use them in the morning, when they will not interfere with your night's sleep. (Caffeine is present in chocolate, coffee, tea, colas and other soft drinks.)

Drinking   If you are going to drink alcohol, do it before 7 P.M. While alcohol is a sedative, it does not lead to restful, productive sleep. Drinking wine with dinner may even prevent you from enjoying a good night's sleep.

Your Roommate   If you share the room with another person, that person's habits may be disturbing your sleep. If you have negative feelings about this person, be he or she a spouse, lover, or someone assigned to you by the dean of students, these feelings could be disturbing your sleep. Perhaps honest communication is needed.

Making Love   If making love relaxes you, before sleep time is a good time for it. If it doesn't, negotiate for another time.

Avoid Tossing and Turning   If you find that you are awake for ten minutes or more, get up. Go to another room and do something not very exciting, like reading the dictionary. Another way to invite sleep to return is to try paradoxical action: when insomnia strikes, get up, sit in a chair, and try to stay awake. Chances are you will become sleepy from the boredom of it all.

The Sleeping Pill Trap   Sleeping medications seldom work on a permanent basis and often can cause a sleep problem. Instead of taking drugs, go to the root of your problem and change whatever it is in your life that is keeping you from sleeping. Your insomnia may be telling you something that numbing yourself may only make worse. If you are already addicted to sleep medications, get help in shaking the problem.

Taking Serious Action   If the cause of your insomnia is related to physical problems that need treatment (like a chemical imbalance or thyroid deficiency), seek medical treatment. If your insomnia came on after a troubling event, such as a death or divorce, or feels like anxiety or depression, get help.

Expanding the Day

Who hasn't fantasized about having more hours in the day? If you are not among the one in three Americans[19] who is trying to get to sleep at night, you are probably thinking wistfully how nice it would be to enjoy more waking hours by sleeping less. For those who want more hours in the day, the obvious place to steal these hours is from sleep time. Yet few of us who try to do it this way succeed. When our bedtime arrives, we forget our resolve and fall asleep.

There are some people who, like elephants, can get by on less than two hours,[20] but they are rare and seem to be born with a different biological clock than the rest of us. The few studies that have been performed on these extremely short sleepers yield that these people appear to have several things in common: they seem to be efficient about their sleeping, falling asleep immediately, then passing through the preliminary stages of sleep quickly; they go right to the stage where the important sleep occurs; and when they are not sleeping, they are active, vigorous, and restless. They also seem to share similar brain-wave patterns.

Becoming one of this group who need only two or three hours of sleep a night is probably not possible for most of us, but we can learn from the sleep researchers to sleep better and to make our own sleeping patterns work for us in ways that will leave us alert and refreshed in the morning. Some of us may be able to learn to become shorter sleepers; without changing our life-style, however, it's unlikely we can vary greatly the time we habitually sleep.

Even short sleepers (those who awaken refreshed after only four to six hours of sleep) live differently from those who sleep longer, said sleep researcher Dr. Ernest Hartmann, who observed that the difference between long and short sleepers, (not the extremely short two-hour sleepers) is their life-style.[21] Dr. Hartmann claims that short sleepers are more likely to be non-worriers. They tend to be active and busy people who do not spend a lot of time thinking about their problems. The long sleepers, by contrast, are more likely to worry and seem to need the restorative values of sleep more than the short sleepers.

Sleeping Less, Living More

A number of the high-energy people I interviewed reported that they sleep very little, but most said they were born sleeping short hours, so they don't know how to explain how they do it. Psychotherapist and professor Loretta Lewis is one of the few in my experience who has deliberately changed from a low-energy, long, restless sleeper to a high-energy short sleeper and has sustained the new regimen for years. Loretta explains how she did it.[22]

"I was very deenergized for many years and slept from 8 to 10 hours a night. I went to bed early, got up late, and never felt totally rested. I realized that my tensions and my stresses were coming from my inability to stop and regenerate myself for a few minutes during the day. So that's what I do. If I stop, relax, and meditate at lunch time, I feel more alive for the rest of the work day. This enables me to function on a higher level." Now Loretta repeats this one other time during the workday and before dinner. "Another change I made was not eating immediately when I got home from work. Instead I did some meditation. Afterward, I was able to relax, enjoy my meal, and not rush and stress myself with things that would irritate me or drain my energy.

"This started about five or six years ago, when I discovered that my body felt very stressed during the day. I went to Silva Mind Control, where I learned to start feeling positive about my body. The more I could be positive about it, the more I became aware of how I was not taking care of myself, which parts of my body I was neglecting, what emotions were really playing havoc with me, and which old anxieties and stresses needed attention. So I focused in on those areas. Soon I began to feel very much alive.

"When I started spending an hour or a little more relaxing and meditating during the day, I found I needed less sleep. Now I can go to sleep at one o'clock and am up by five, which gives me four hours' sleep. My body feels very different. When I awaken I feel rested, energized, and am very relaxed. I can do all those things that I missed for all the years when I was totally drained and would fall asleep at ten or ten-thirty."

It could be argued that Loretta is substituting meditation time for sleep time. Loretta responds: "Before, my energy was so drained that I couldn't enjoy anything. One reason was because of my fear that I wouldn't get enough sleep. Now I feel as though I am living a full day. I have at least five extra hours each day to spend on enjoyment. I am not taking that time and energy and doing a lot of work with it, but I'm doing a lot of pleasurable things, which enhances my energy. I've found that the more pleasurable things that I do with the extra time that I have, the more energy I get and the less sleep I need."

Worry, stress, and the need to sleep seem to be related in yet unknown ways. A life change to alleviate worry and stress, like the regular meditation practice Loretta implemented, can affect sleep needs. It's probably no coincidence that advanced yogis (who meditate a lot) need to sleep very little.

Research conducted at the Himalayan Institute, a training, research, and rehabilitation center in Honesdale, Pennsylvania, shows that breathing training followed by physical hatha yoga significantly improved people's moods and reduced their need for sleep. The researchers also found that the simple practice of diaphragmatic breathing (see Step 1) *without* the physical exercise of hatha created a significant change in the emotional levels of mood and anxiety. It also reduced the need for sleep.[23]

Step 3.   Energizing Food

Like everyone else, I resist changing my eating habits. I hold style of eating, along with the ballot box and religion, to be basic personal freedoms, so I don't want to proselytize about food. The information given here is not meant to be another diet, but a way to make better food choices.

Most of us already know how to eat better than we do. But we're busy people and it's easy to resist thinking about eating better. In our nation of riches and natural abundance, along with our high literacy rate, we should be the healthiest, longest-living people that ever walked the earth. We're not — but we could be — if living well, long and energetically were higher on our list of collective priorities.

Since there's no one between us and our forks to take

this responsibility, that leaves you and me — the captains of our own ships and chefs in our own kitchens! We're in charge here, so let's be informed.[24]

Your Heart and Your Energy

Scenario: There's a good chance that the last time you had a checkup, you were told about your blood serum cholesterol count in general terms like "okay" or "medium" or "average." So you didn't ask any more questions, because you felt safe and secure.

Cholesterol, a soapy, fatty substance, is essential to life. Our bodies use it to manufacture and maintain heathy cells. While we make most of the cholesterol ourselves, some of it comes from our foods.

A serum cholesterol count measures the different kinds and amounts of cholesterol circulating in the bloodstream. The cholesterol is bound to lipoproteins and is carried by them. These fatty compounds can clump together and constrict the blood flow in the arteries around the heart, causing heart disease.

The two kinds of lipoproteins we hear the most about are H.D.L. (high-density lipoproteins) and L.D.L. (low-density lipoproteins). The H.D.L.'s are beneficial, the L.D.L.'s are the ones that cause trouble (which is why some people call them "Little Devils.")

Most of us (except for a small minority who have a hereditary tendency toward high serum cholesterol) can reduce the amount of serum cholesterol circulating in the bloodstream by exercising, practicing deep relaxation, and making prudent food choices. A high blood serum cholesterol count is a warning sign that we are not living in harmony with our bodies' needs. Heeding this warning and learning to live differently is life-saving as well as energy-enhancing (because healthy arteries allow more oxygen to be delivered to the tissues).

Are you informed of the health of your arteries? Do you know your blood serum cholesterol count? Until recently many physicians considered heart disease a normal part of the aging process and tended to tell their patients that as long as their blood serum cholesterol level was under 250 (or, in some cases, between 200 and 300), they were "okay" or "average." In 1985 both my father and my husband were told by different doctors that they were average or low average when their serum cholesterol levels were in the 240-250 range. Because both read the word *average* to mean *safe*, both interpreted this statement as an assurance that gave them a false sense of security. But blood serum cholesterol counts of 240 and 250 are not safe.

It is true that because so many Americans are in this range, a reading of 250 is indeed "average." Yet half of the heart attack victims are within the low medium or average range, so average doesn't mean safe.[25]

Heart disease is epidemic in America. Who wants to have "average" chances in an epidemic?

I don't. Not when there's something I can do to improve my risk factor, and there's a lot I can do. For most of us, our risk factor for heart disease is something that we can alter on our own, without drugs.

I asked Dr. William Castelli about this. Dr. Castelli is the director of the Framingham Heart Study, the longest-running (nearly forty years) study and most comprehensive project of its kind. He replied, "This is one of the biggest errors that continues in American medicine today. Many physicians treat only those patients in the top 10% — those at highest risk. Half the heart attack victims in America have cholesterol levels between 150 and 250, but because their total serum cholesterol count is under 250, they are being completely ignored by physicians."

Dr. Castelli recommends being knowledgeable about the health of your arteries, learning not only the exact number of the serum cholesterol count, but other calculations as well. He says, "The single best predictor we have of whether a person will have a future heart attack is the ratio of total cholesterol to H.D.L. cholesterol. Yet this simple calculation is not routinely done. We doctors are not treating the easiest group to treat!"

This ratio is determined by dividing the total cholesterol by the beneficial H.D.L. cholesterol. Dr. Castelli recommends that anyone whose ratio of total cholesterol to H.D.L. cholesterol is higher than 4.5:1 should be treated to lower that ratio. Ask your doctor to check this.

Better yet, get your total serum cholesterol count down to 150. Statistically, people with total serum cholesterol counts that low are in a very low-risk category for heart attacks. (*Keeping* the count low is the important part. Your total serum cholesterol count is really a reflection of how you lived for the last three to twenty-eight days. To change *risk* categories, it is necessary to maintain a lower count for two or three years.)[26]

Dr. Castelli says, "If your cholesterol level is under 150, you are not going to have a heart attack — even if you smoke, have hypertension, and everything else."[27]

I haven't achieved a score of 150 yet, but my 162 is a big improvement over the 225-plus serum cholesterol counts that I had before I started living the Energistics way.

Does your doctor take the time to explain things like this to you? Or do you avoid asking questions because you don't want to appear stupid? Following are some intelligent questions to ask your doctor when you receive the results of your blood serum cholesterol tests:

- What is the total serum cholesterol count? (Ask for numbers, not generalizations.)
- What is the count of high-density lipoproteins?
- What is the ratio of total cholesterol to H.D.L. cholesterol? (You can figure this out if you have the numbers mentioned previously.)
- What does this result mean?
- What can be done to improve this ratio?
- Is the total blood serum cholesterol count in the range in which heart attacks and strokes frequently happen?
- What can be done to lower this figure to a safer level?

Learn to be a knowledgeable health consumer. Love your heart enough to give it your active attention. Take the responsibility for your own well-being and make an appointment to have your blood serum cholesterol tested today. Do it right by fasting for twelve hours before the test and abstaining from alcohol for twenty-four hours. Then ask questions.

Are Vegetarians Really Healthier?

Most of us don't want to be reminded that we are making life-and-death decisions every time we pick up a fork. But energists and lovers of life won't settle for this head-in-the-sand approach. Fortunately, knowing how to make intelligent food choices has become easier in the last few years because there is more agreement among the experts.

Most seem to recommend that we aim for a low-fat, high-fiber menu, — that is, lower fat and higher fiber than what we as a nation are now eating. Although the experts differ on what they think we can accomplish in the way of change, there is little serious disagreement on what would be best for us.

It's hard to argue with substantial research that concludes vegetarians are the healthiest group and live the longest, and I urge you to consider this choice. But because the nutritional and medical experts are being realistic about how fast and how much we are willing to change, they are recommending instead a sort of semi-vegetarian diet.

The term accurately discribes my own menu choices. I choose most of my foods from the vegetable group, with the addition of fish and dairy products. A study of restaurant menus convinces me that this is an increasingly popular trend. However, the term does not mean complete abstinence from meat. This is an important distinction.

A few definitions are in order here. A *vegan* is a strict vegetarian who eats foods of plant origin only. A *lacto-ovo-vegetarian* consumes milk, and eggs, but no fish, meat, or poultry. (Most U.S. vegetarians are in this category.) A *semi-vegetarian* thinks of meat as a flavoring for other foods. Included in this category are those who eat as lacto-ovo-vegetarians at home, but eat whatever is served in the homes of others.

All of us can lower our risk factors by eating more like the vegetarians, even if we do not strictly limit ourselves. But some of my meat-loving friends have told me they don't believe they could be healthy on a vegetarian regimen or anything resembling one. Let's look at how strict vegetarians fare in recent research:

- *The Journal of the American Medical Association* reported that a vegetarian diet tends to lower the blood pressure; a meat diet tends to raise it.[28]

- An article in *Obstretrics & Gynecology* stated that women who eat more animal fat tend to get more ovarian cancer than women who eat a smaller amount of animal fat.[29]

- The same source said that vegetarians tend to be leaner.[30]

- Another source stated that vegetarians are less prone to bone-density loss. Loss of bone density leads to brittle bones, back problems.[31]

- Vegetarians have lower blood serum cholesterol levels than meat eaters, but these levels rise when only eight ounces of meat is added daily for one month, stated *The Journal of Human Nutrition*.[32]

- Vegetarian women have considerably less pollutant chemicals in their breast milk (and presumably, in themselves,) than do meat eaters, wrote *The New York Times*.[33]

- In a ten-year study of seven thousand men, those who had heart attacks tended to chose foods that contained more protein and fats than men who choose food that contained more carbohydrates. In addition, those who died of their heart attacks had consistently chosen more protein and fats than those who survived.[34]

- Vegetarians in the Framingham Heart Study were, as a group, more likely to have lower blood fat levels than meat eaters.[35] In addition, they had more H.D.L. (the good kind of cholesterol) in their blood than a presumably healthy group of Boston Marathon runners (who were also physicians).

Some researchers have expressed concern that a very low cholesterol count may predispose an individual to certain forms of cancer, so I asked Dr. William Castelli of the Framingham Heart Study whether it is dangerous to allow our cholesterol levels to become too low. "Absolutely not," says Dr. Castelli. "The vegetarians have the lowest cholesterol counts, the lowest rates of cancer and heart disease."[36] He continued, referring to current data from the Framingham Heart Study, "Of those with a total cholesterol count less than 180, more are alive today. Those with the lowest cholesterol levels have outlived everyone else."

Sorry, devoted carnivores. Vegetarians seem to be the healthiest group of people. And to the resistant who claims that "Humans are designed to be meat eaters! The way out teeth are shaped proves that our ancestors were meat eaters!" I reply that it's worth remembering they didn't just drive down to the supermarket for a steak, but had to chase it through the forest (thereby lowering cholesterol) and they probably didn't catch it every day. Between successful hunts, they ate such things as high-fiber fruits and grains.

Our jaws aren't the only evidence of our genetic predilection. Our taste buds naturally attract us to sweets (like berries and starches), and the length of our intestinal tract indicates that we are well-adapted to be herbivores.

If we could eat in the style of our ancestors, maybe we could be healthy on a largely meat-inclusive diet. After all, the meat available to them was simply not like what we eat today. A commercially raised steer may be 30% fat. Even today, wild meat has far less, maybe only 4% fat or less, and doesn't contain antibiotics or artificial hormones.

It may not be necessary to abstain completely from meat and other animal foods in order to gain many of the health benefits associated with vegetarianism. The next few sections tell you how.

How to Gain the Vegetarian Advantage (Without Going All the Way)

What the vegetarians don't eat gets most of the attention, yet it's probably as important from a health perspective to discover what they *do* eat that makes them so healthy.

First, they eat more fruit, vegetables and grains, which

automatically include the healthful fibers. Second, they probably eat less fat, but certainly less of the saturated, animal-based fats. This agrees with what nutritional experts are telling us: The most important change most of us can make is to eat less fat, especially that of animal origin. Some are more emphatic and say that the typical American diet contains too much animal fat and is downright dangerous.

In a typical U.S. daily menu, up to 45% of the calories are fat and 25% are sugar. That leaves only about 30% for real food — the kind that meets your additional requirements for protein, vitamins, minerals, and fibers![37] It's no wonder that Americans are overfed and underenergized.

Dr. Oliver Alabaster, director of cancer research at George Washington University, writes: "Up to 60% of cancer can be prevented with diet alone!" He claims that our traditional high-fat diet is one of the factors that encourages cancer.[38]

Some fat in the diet is necessary and desirable, but the experts differ about what percentage of total calories in fats would be ideal. However, they agree on this: Whatever we can do as individuals to get ourselves out of the high-risk group for heart disease, strokes, and cancer is the right thing to do.

Health organizations (including the American Heart Association) have recommended that fat intake be cut to 30% of the total calories. (Oils count as fats.) Of course, if your fat intake is already lower than 30%, no one is suggesting that you raise it! Judging from countries that have a lower incidence of heart disease, it seems that a fat intake between 10% and 20% would be a lot better.

Those who recommend 30% and under are very specific about which fats to use. They suggest dividing your daily intake of 30% into three parts: $^1/_3$ polyunsaturated fat in the form of corn or safflower oil, $^1/_3$ saturated fat from animal sources, and $^1/_3$ monounsaturated fat from olive or peanut oil.[39]

These recommendations are good to keep in mind when choosing food, but, in fact, most of us won't weigh and measure what we eat. My system is simpler. I use the smallest amount of fat required to make food palatable, avoiding saturated fats as much as possible. I like my food to taste good, and it takes only a tiny bit of fat (certainly less than 30%) to bring out the flavor.

When I need to add a fat to a food, I usually use olive oil. Unlike the newly developed oils, olive oil has been around for 6000 years, and researchers still haven't found anything wrong with it. It's rich in monounsaturated fatty acids, which have been shown to be beneficial in reducing total serum cholesterol.[40] Although this is not yet conclusive, new studies suggest that a diet rich in monounsaturated fatty acids appears to be at least as effective in lowering plasma cholesterol as a diet low in fat and high in carbohydrates.[41] This is good news because foods containing olive oil can be much more interesting than those containing little or no fat.

Another plus for olive oil is that it resists becoming rancid and doesn't need to be refrigerated. Peanut and sesame oils are all right, too.

I use very little of the polyunsaturated oils, limiting them to baked goods (which wouldn't taste right made with olive oil). The polyunsaturates (safflower oil, corn oils) also reduce serum cholesterol, but there is some suspicion that these may, in large amounts, be a factor in the development of cancer.

Of the saturated fats, I use the smallest amounts I can manage, while maintaining a great variety in my menus. The following are suggestions for ways to reduce your consumption of fats:

- If you use meat, make it a minor — not a major — part of the food on your plate. When there is a choice between white and red meat, go for the white. Always cut off the fat, and remove the skin on poultry. Skim the fat off homemade soups by refrigerating before serving.
- Notice the grease that accumulates in the pan when meat containing fat has been cooked. After it has cooled a bit, take a good long look at it. Is this what you want clogging up your arteries, depriving you of oxygen?
- If you eat meat, chicken is considered a "better" choice, but beware of fast-food chicken. Researchers at the Center for Science in the Public Interest report that eight of the largest fast-food chains cook French fries and other foods in beef tallow, which is high in saturated fats. If you order a chicken sandwich — on the premise that chicken should be relatively healthful — it may be deep-fried in this tallow and have the equivalent fat and cholesterol of 11 pats of butter![42]
- Beware of fast food in general. A typical

meal at a popular fast-food restaurant chain consisting of a double cheeseburger, fries, and a shake contains 1,410 milligrams of sodium, 10 teaspoons of sugar, and 21 teaspoons of fat! That's almost ½ cup of fat![43] Anything containing this much fat should include a surgeon general's warning: "Eating this could be hazardous to your health!"

- Use only low- or no-fat dairy products. One or 2% milk sounds like a tiny amount of fat, but when you remove the water from your calculations, 1% or low-fat milk contains 24% fat![44] Avoid sour cream by substituting low-fat yogurt. Spread butter thinly and work toward getting along without it altogether.

- Margarine is made of hydrogenated polyunsaturated oil. Although it is of plant origin, after being hydrogenated (to make the product hard at room temperature) some of the oil becomes saturated, which is not good for your heart. In addition, it contains many additives. This whole process makes it an unnatural, synthetic food. Some experts believe that margarine may be worse for the heart than butter. If you do use margarine, buy only the kind that lists *liquid* polyunsaturated oil as the first ingredient. Avoid those that are made with palm oil, coconut oil, or lard. Palm and coconut oils are very saturated fats, even though they are liquid at room temperature. Beware of a product called "popcorn oil," which is made from these cheaper oils.

- Our family has discovered that really good fresh bread doesn't need any spread at all. Search for good, grainy bread. Better yet, make your own (only if you enjoy it) or barter with a friend who does. De-vitalized white bread invites fat gooey toppings and uses space in your menu that you could devote to better things — like fiber.

- Low-fat foods seem somewhat bland until we learn to taste in a new way. Since fat "carries the flavor," one solution is to add lots of flavor. I mean *lots* more. Discover the joys of lemon, onions, horseradish, herbs, garlic, green chilies, flavored vinegars, exotic mustards, red, black, and white pepper. (Garlic contains a substance that reduces serum cholesterol in animals and probably in us as well.)[45]

A sensible, middle-of-the-road approach would be to reduce the fats you ingest now by switching to those of vegetable origin. When you get used to this way of eating, you may be able to reduce the fat level further and still enjoy your food. What surprised me was that recipes I used years ago when I ate more fats and oils now seem unpleasantly heavy.

Eating is one of life's great pleasures. Don't pass it by. But do check your progress with regular cholesterol counts. Try to score below 180, or take Dr. Castelli's recommendation and aim for 150.

The Fat-Fiber Connection

Fortunately, eating for health and energy isn't only a matter of "Thou shalt nots." Let's add one healthful imperative to our daily menu planning: "Thou shalt eat fiber."

Dr. James Anderson of the University of Kentucky Medical College linked eating some kinds of fiber with the lowering of blood levels of cholesterol. He reported successful results in lowering the serum cholesterol count of people with high counts by having them eat several oat-bran muffins a day.[46]

Dr. Kenneth Storch of the Massachusetts Institute of Technology used healthy students as subjects to test Dr. Anderson's hypothesis. He had one group eat four wheat-bran muffins a day and another group eat four oat-bran muffins a day in addition to regular college food. Those who ate wheat-bran muffins showed no drop in cholesterol, while those who ate oat-bran muffins showed a total reduction of 5% within two weeks. Dr. Storch says, "Such a drop in cholesterol levels means a 10% drop in the chances of a person having a heart attack."

It sounds too good to be true. Does this mean that we can eat unlimited fats as long as we eat plenty of oat-bran muffins? Probably not. It may mean that by including exercise, relaxation, and "positive foods" like oat bran in one's daily life, some people will be able to rely more on foods and less upon drugs for cholesterol reduction.

To lower my husband's serum cholesterol count, we used a variation of Dr. Anderson's idea. We mixed oat bran with our morning hot cereal, baked it into cookies and muffins, and reduced the level of fat in the family dinners. My husband cut back on eating egg yolks, and he paid a little more attention to the food he ate away from home (where he eats about 40% of the time). His serum cholesterol level decreased from 243 to 176 in two short months! (My husband is also a runner, which may be part of the reason for these dramatic results.)

Researchers A. A. Qureshi, W. C. Burger, and colleagues at the University of Wisconsin studied the fiber-cholesterol connection by feeding animals diets of different grains. They learned that serum cholesterol could be reduced as much as 18% depending upon the grain used. On the animals tested, barley worked the best, said Dr. Burger, with oats, rye, and wheat following respectively. Corn and rice did not work nearly as well.[47]

The Wisconsin researchers explained that it is not the crudeness of the fiber itself that lowers the cholesterol, but several substances found in the fibrous part of these particular grains. Dr. Qureshi says these substances are found in a wide variety of common, unrefined foods, and that we will get enough of them if we decrease our meat portions and choose from a wide range of whole unprocessed foods, including the two superstars, oats and barley.

The grains that do not reduce your cholesterol count (wheat, corn, rice) still deserve a place at your table. Some fibers (like wheat bran) absorb water, increasing stool bulk and causing a laxative effect. Moving the food through the body more rapidly may provide protection from certain gastric and intestinal cancers and sometimes can give a perceptible energy boost to those with sluggish digestive systems.

Certain vegetable fibers contain substances that have

been shown to reduce specific cancer risks, particularly of the stomach and bowels. In addition to avoiding fats, experts recommend the protective fibers found in whole grains, citrus fruits and vegetables, especially the cruciferous vegetables (broccoli, Brussels sprouts, cabbage.)[48] Including more calcium-rich foods (skim milk, buttermilk, etc.) increases this protection as well.[49]

If you are on a prescribed diet or medication, please don't alter this without consulting your physician. But consider discussing these possibilities at your next checkup. Many people prefer to be given a pill rather than be told about things like fiber and exercise. Let your medical advisor know where *you* stand.

I asked Dr. Qureshi whether it is possible that eating great quantities of unrefined foods might be unhealthy. "Nature provides the balance," he said, "as long as you use the whole food." Therefore, choose the *whole* grain over processed; the *whole* fruit over pasteurized, filtered juice; and the *whole* vegetable (minus husks and other inedible parts). And Dr. Qureshi makes another good point: Exercise moderation in food choices.

How to Add Fiber

Processing food removes much of the natural fiber, as well as needed nutrients. This process also includes the addition of artificial additives your body doesn't need. The colorful packaging increases the price. So when you treat your body to a natural food, as close as possible to the way it occurred in nature on root, branch, stalk, or vine, you are doing more for yourself than including natural fiber. In addition, by choosing vegetable-based foods close to their natural state, you are probably avoiding a lot of calorie-laden fat (unless you are fond of smothering your food in butter, cheese, or hollandaise sauce), so you can eat more.

Apricots, spinach, raspberries, cabbage, kale, okra, asparagus, and broccoli are all good sources of fiber and are wonderful foods. (If you buy them in season, you'll get another benefit: a lower price.) How long has it been since you've tasted a hearty bean soup? Fiber-filled dried legumes like lentils, pintos, and black beans are always available and always a bargain. Pound for pound, nutrient for nutrient, plant-based natural foods cost less than meat or packaged, refined foods.

Some obvious substitutions: brown rice for instant rice; real potatoes for boxed ones; fresh or frozen vegetables instead of canned. In its kernel form, barley can be used as a substitute for rice or pasta (barley casserole, barley soup, marinated barley salad with scallions and carrots). Whatever grain you use, be it barley, oats, rye, or wheat, use the whole grain whenever you can. The refined grains — quick-cooking rice, quick-cooking oatmeal, and pour-and-serve oatmeal products — have had most of the healthful ingredients removed.

Whole grains take longer to cook, but you don't have to stand by the stove and watch them. If you set the timer, you can do something else (like exercise).

"White food" (made with white flour and sugar) does little except increase your size and tickle your tongue. Don't be fooled by hidden white food that has been dyed some other color, such as brown, to make it look like whole wheat. (Exceptions to this are milk, potatoes, and cauliflower, which are naturally white.) Gradually replace devitalized foods in your daily menu with the real thing.

Don't confuse the word *cellulose* with fiber. Some low-calorie breads labeled "diet" or "lite" list an ingredient called *alpha-cellulose*. Most of these products reduce the calories by adding indigestible wood pulp, which may or may not be beneficial.

Eating what nature offers in the form that food most naturally occurs is what our bodies require for healthful and energetic living. Natural eating is the way we cooperate with our design. The world is full of enough conflict, I believe, without battling our biology at the table.

Kissing Bacon Good-bye — Slowly

Eating for health and energy may be a whole new way of thinking about food, but it's not a good idea to begin with any idea of deprivation. If you are accustomed to eating a lot of meat, please regard my suggestions as an expansion in culinary possibilities, a broadening of your horizons. The way to make room in your menu for a greater variety of delicious and healthy foods is to decrease the fat. Most of the fat comes with the meat, so eating a larger proportion of food from vegetable sources almost certainly will lower your fat consumption, particularly your consumption of saturated fat.

A person who reduces the fat level in the daily menu often begins to feel lighter and more energetic after meals. This is because fat requires more oxygen to digest. Another bonus: eating meat becomes less desirable, and vegetables you never noticed before start to taste really good. By gradually adding low-fat, vegetable-based foods that you truly like, you can almost painlessly ease out some of the common heart-busters like fatty meat, gravy, and butter.

When you decide to incorporate some of these suggestions into your eating habits, beware of making big changes all at once. Adding a large amount of fiber suddenly may cause gas, create an uncomfortable feeling, make you discouraged, or interfere with your absorption of vitamins. If you proceed gradually and include a great variety of foods, this is not likely to be a problem. You will not only ease the adjustment, you will also keep peace in the family. It takes tact, patience, and compromise to change a family's eating habits. Schedule the transition over years, not weeks.

If you are the meal planner, first adjust to the idea that every meal does not have to be based upon an animal food. This requires some conscious decisions — and some new cookbooks. How to make the transition? Cook a couple of meals from a good vegetarian cookbook one or two days a week. On alternate days create dishes in which meat is a small part, a featured flavoring rather than the bulk of the meal. Next month serve the same dish without the meat. Or make a big vegetable-and-pasta entrée and serve meat as a side dish. Next month put a protein-rich vegetable into the same pasta recipe and skip the meat side dish. Serve your regular menus in between.

It takes a while to become skilled at new kinds of cooking. Give yourself time. There is an immense variety of non-animal based foods. The magazine *Vegetarian Times* offers delicious suggestions.[50] There are many good cookbooks, and opportunities to take classes in various kinds of ethnic vegetarian cooking abound.

I hope you will take the following "Relative Goodness" list as a guideline, a way to be informed about making dietary changes. Too many rules make for a rigid life. As long as you want to eat meat, eat some. Your body will tell you when it's ready for a change. Remember that it is what you do every day that counts, not an occasional nibble that will do you in. If you have a wild craving for something, at least enjoy the transgression. Don't waste energy on self-flagellation. The guilt will do you more harm than occasionally giving in to those impulses. Enjoy your food and be good to yourself.

Tune in to yourself instead. Eventually, your body will tell you when you feed it something that isn't healthful. Before you reach for an antacid pill or a laxative, say to yourself, "What is it my body is trying to tell me with this discomfort?" When you become sensitive to your body's language, your body will lead you to better choices. If you have been eating a steady diet of junk foods, your body's ability to communicate is probably skewed. You may consciously have to give it better treatment before you can trust the messages. Even one piece of rich dessert or fat-laden meat will produce an uncomfortable feeling for most people who have been eating only optimal foods for a while. Bless the feeling. That's your body talking.

Remember: It wouldn't be wise to go "cold turkey." Instead, add an artichoke here, a handful of beans there. If you want to make permanent changes and still keep peace in your family, you should move at a snail's pace.

The "Relative Goodness" Food List

Being a semi-vegetarian doesn't mean existing on nuts, seeds, and a few green stalks. This is not a new diet, but a new emphasis, a new way to look at the same old dinner plate.

To simplify the information in the last few sections, I have summarized it in a list. This is for you to use in determining the relative goodness of various foods — from the best to the worst — based upon recent research findings.

****ANYTIME — Choose most of your foods from this group (these are preferred foods for building health and energy):

- Most fruits and vegetables and real, unsweetened juices
- Whole grains and whole-grain products (bread, cereals, pasta)
- Dried beans and peas
- White and sweet potatoes
- Flavor vegetables and derivatives like garlic, onions, horseradish, mustard, flavored vinegars
- Skim milk and cultured skim-milk products (cottage cheese, buttermilk)
- Egg whites only

***THE FOLLOWING ARE GOOD FOODS WHEN USED IN PROPORTIONALLY SMALLER QUANTITIES THAN THE PRECEDING 4-STAR LIST:

- Fresh seafood and fish
- Lean meats, like turkey and chicken
- Canned or frozen fish (fresh is better)
- Salad oils (see explanation of oils)
- Nuts, seeds (in main dishes, not as roasted and salted snacks)
- Low-fat milk products (such as cottage cheese, yogurt.

**THE "ONCE IN A WHILE" LIST:

- Egg yolks
- Ice cream
- Hard cheeses and products made with cheese (like cheesecake)
- Red meat (only if you really like it)
- Smoked fish
- Butter
- White-flour products
- White rice
- Bagels
- Avocado

*THE "ALMOST NEVER" LIST (These have little nutritional value and it is easy to find better substitutions; If you don't eat these for a while, they cease to seem attractive):

- Soup mixes
- Coffee whiteners
- Sugar
- Soda

- Coffee
- Chocolate
- Pastries
- Bacon, sausages and other preserved meats
- Salted nuts
- Potato chips and other salted snack foods
- Added salt
- Artificial sweeteners
- Artificial dessert toppings
- Lard and meat fat
- Deep-fried foods

(NOTE: This list is offered for your convenience and with the assumption that you have no allergies or other special needs.)

Explore the joys of many foods and eat them as close to the way nature presents them as possible. By making wiser food choices, you may soon start feeling more energetic.

Eating Out

Restaurants are responding to the trend toward lighter eating. You may see "Dine to Your Heart's Content" printed on the menu. Some restaurants use terms like "Spa Cuisine" and "Light and Lively" to indicate low-fat selections. Most good restaurants can prepare a low-fat meal for you if you call ahead. Even carry-out delicatessens are offering lighter food. Banquet caterers will substitute fish or vegetable plates for high-calorie, high-fat, meat-based entrées if you let them know ahead. Most airlines will provide vegetarian, low-fat or low-cholesterol menus. Make your food request when you book your reservation.

Being a guest in someone's home *after* you have decided to eat lighter food is a different situation. Eating differently tends to separate people, and hosts easily can be offended. A generous helping of tact, seasoned with a little humor, will be appreciated.

Today most people understand if you prefer salad rather than steak with your baked potato. But a meal shared with people I care about is special, and I want my hosts to feel relaxed and comfortable. Being fussy about food someone has generously offered is in bad form and wholly unnecessary. I follow the advice of W. S. Gilbert, who wrote: "It isn't so much what's on the table that matters, as what's on the chairs."

The Energist's Breakfast

What did you have for breakfast today? Eggs and bacon? Cold cereal? Nothing at all?

The usual American breakfast consisting of "eat and run" doesn't build health or energy. But what are the better choices? Eggs with yolks are a no-no for many now. Cold cereal made of once-healthful grain has been processed to lifelessness and embalmed with artificial additives. (From the viewpoint of pure kitchen economics, boxed cereals are not bargains. Grind the contents of one of those big cereal boxes in a food processor to see how much air you have paid for. Nutrient for nutrient, ounce for ounce, hot cereal is much less expensive.) Some cold cereals hidden under a lot of milk or yogurt and fruit may be a filling snack, but this is hardly an energy-enhancing way to start the day.

So what's left? Hot cereal. Not the old gooey kind that the college cafeteria had on a steam table all week but a delicious twenty-first-century, full-energy breakfast, consisting of an almost infinite variety of grain and fruit combinations.

I can hear you saying, "Where can I find the time to make a full-energy breakfast?" By using the time while the grains are cooking to do something else. (It's not necessary to stand there and watch it cook!) If I have forty-five minutes I make barley or brown rice and do forty-two minutes of hatha. Those with young children can start the grains cooking immediately upon arising and then get everyone ready. If forty-five minutes is longer than you can spend on these other preparations, there are quicker cereal grains. Millet takes twenty minutes. Bulghur (cracked wheat) is easy because you put the grains in boiling water, cover, and turn off the heat. In fifteen minutes it has cooked itself.

Or try old-fashioned oatmeal. It's high in protein and fiber, contains no added fat, and cooks in 5 minutes — about the same time it takes to pack lunches.

Although I prefer to use whole grains, in a pinch I'll make cooked bran, which boils up faster than I can set the table. My friend Mary Longtine's Super Fiber Invention (1/2 wheat bran and 1/2 oat bran, plus lots of fruit) takes less than 1 minute to cook once the fruit is cut and the water is boiling. The fastest but not the tastiest cereal of all is plain, cooked oat bran, which takes about

30 seconds at my altitude. I can make that faster than I could find all the ingredients for cold cereal (which would leave me feeling like I hadn't eaten).

If you are not awake enough to cook in the morning, you can use plain leftover millet, buckwheat, bulghur, or brown rice from dinner. These can be fixed almost instantly in the morning, either by reheating on the stove (with more liquid) or for forty seconds in the microwave. Add fruit, of course. Experiment before you give up. A good breakfast will keep your energy sparkling all day.

How to Be a Morning Gourmet

I can hear you saying, "Hot cereal? Yuk!" I used to think so, too, until my sister introduced me to Gourmet Oatmeal and Goldilocks Porridge. Now elegant cooked-cereal breakfasts are one of my specialties, and I often have my morning yoga class in for breakfast to prove it. They actually like it.

What sets this cereal apart is fruit — *lots* of fruit. I add whatever is in season: apples, bananas, peaches, kiwis, along with seeds, nuts, currants, or raisins, *while the oatmeal, rice, millet, or whatever grain is cooking*, until I have put in about 50% "extras." Cooked bananas? — I add 1/2 to 1 whole banana for every serving. You have to try it to believe it. I end up with a delicious concoction that is more of a fruity pudding than the usual wallpaper paste in a bowl with fruit on top. If you add enough fruits and nuts, you won't need sweetening, but honey or maple syrup (salt if you must) enhances it.

The recipe changes with the availability of seasonal fruit. Try our current favorite before you decide that "Gourmet Oatmeal" is a contradiction in terms. It tastes rather like apple-pie filling.

Gourmet Oatmeal

Turn on the burner. Pour 2 cups of water and 1 cup of apple juice (or 2 cups of water and 1 cup of skim milk) into a pan with 1 cup of Old-Fashioned Rolled Oats. Slice in 2 bananas and 1 or 2 Granny Smith apples. Toss in a handful of raisins and some almonds or sunflower seeds. (If you're strenuously avoiding fats, skip the nuts and seeds.) Lower the heat, cover, and set the timer for 5 minutes. Add a shake of cinnamon and a few drops of vanilla if you have time. *Makes 3 large servings.*

If you want the cholesterol-lowering protection concentrated in the bran of the oats, use a little less oatmeal than the directions specify. One minute before removing from the heat, stir in enough Quaker Mother's Oat Bran to make the mixture the right consistency. For a maximum cholesterol-reducing breakfast, try barley and add oat bran as above.

More breakfast ideas: (Grains vary, so follow package directions.)

The Piña Colada

Cook brown rice with crushed pineapple and coconut. It's even better when part of the liquid is pineapple juice and skim milk. Allow 40 minutes for the rice to cook.

Goldilocks Porridge

Cook millet 20 minutes with bananas, fresh peaches, and dried currants. If you add chia seeds, you won't be hungry until noon.

The North America

An elegant company breakfast is made by cooking together brown rice and wild rice (3/4 cup of brown rice, 1/4 cup of wild rice, 2 cups of water) for about 40 minutes. When it is done, add toasted pecans and maple syrup. If you are watching your fat intake carefully, save this for special occasions only because pecans contain oil.

Get some good whole grains and express your creativity. Many are available in any grocery store and are the same grains that you would serve later in the day with different seasonings as a main or side dish, so you may have them in your cupboard already. On weekends when there's more time, there are more low-fat breakfast choices: whole-grain pancakes topped with fruit; *frittatas* made with many vegetables and only the whites of the eggs; scrambled tofu; French toast, made with egg whites, orange juice, and cinnamon; and, of course, bran muffins. (When baking, use baking powder that does not contain aluminum, an ingredient that is controversial.)

Most people who are watching their cholesterol eliminate egg yolks entirely. If your doctor suggests a limitation of two egg yolks per week, as many do, you can make these go further by using "half eggs," (one yolk and three whites per serving). Ask your doctor how many egg yolks per week are right for you. (What to do with the extra yolks? Cook them and give them to your dog. My veterinarian tells me that cholesterol build-up is not a problem for dogs.)

And what if you don't eat breakfast, especially not "bird food?" Dr. Asaf Qureshi recommends a glass or two of buttermilk (made from skim milk) for those who won't sit down to a real breakfast. He says he has never seen an elderly woman with "dowager's hump" (a condition caused by calcium loss) in rural villages in India and Pakistan, where breakfasting on buttermilk is the custom. An excellent food, the fat has been removed, but the good things — protein, calcium, "friendly bacteria" — remain. The slightly sour flavor really opens your eyes in the morning.

Time and Optimal Nourishment

Life is full of necessary compromises. Time is important to busy and energetic people. Below are ways to allocate the expenditure of your time more efficiently in areas that build health. Ultimately, better health means more energy, which saves you time.

Budget Time and Make Lists   In a survey by the *New Age Journal*, 73% of the readers identified themselves as "not omnivorous," meaning they eat mostly vegetables. Most stated they spent an hour per day on meal preparation, but many said they accomplished these tasks in ten to twenty minutes.[51]

Plan Ahead   Since the members of my family have unpredictable schedules, I depend upon "planned-overs," to keep the refrigerator full. Example: I soak a whole bag of dried beans one day to cook the next. When they are cooked tender I remove one-third of the beans with a sieved spoon and marinate them with scallions, herbs, olive oil, and vinegar for salad additions later in the week. I remove another one-third of the beans and put them in the food processor (with plenty of seasonings and olive oil) to use as stuffing for enchiladas for that day's dinner. I freeze the leftover enchiladas for quick meals the next week. I freeze or refrigerate the remainder of the beans and broth so I have a head start on soup for the weekend. That's four meals out of one pot, and none are the same. I keep rotating beans and grains and vegetables so that there's always plenty of variety on the table, and in the refrigerator and freezer. Organizing this way cuts cooking time to a fraction and is very economical.

Use Available Help   Children can be enlisted to help in the kitchen and read labels in a grocery store; it's good for them to have some awareness about their food. Let them play detective for excessive salt and sugar content. (Learning to say "no" to certain additives in foods as they grow may make it easier for them to say "no" to other chemicals as teens.)

Read Labels   Ingredients are listed on the label in order of quantity. In many processed foods, sugar heads the list. Avoid these. And beware of sugar called by other names — corn syrup, glucose, lactose. Sugar is a devitalized non-food that can cause fatigue, depression, and lack of concentration. This may be because it replaces needed nutrients in the diet or because the symptoms indicate that there is a problem in metabolizing sugar. Do you crave sugar? See your doctor and ask for a five-hour glucose test.

Salt   Sodium is a necessary nutrient, but most of us

consume too much. Excess sodium has been linked to problems such as high blood pressure and edema. Most processed foods contain an overabundance of salt. Avoid anything with sodium in its name, like monosodium glutamate. Sodium nitrate is linked to cancer in laboratory animals. You would want to avoid this preservative anyway, because it occurs in meat products that are too high in fat.

Out of Sight/Out of Mind The best time to do your food selection is in the grocery store, not at the table. Think twice before you bring anything into your house that does not build health. (This is particularly challenging when you have children who have been conditioned by advertising to want "television foods.") When you are in the process of changing to better eating habits, stock up on appetizing, healthful snacks. Keep fresh fruits and vegetables and "better snacks" ready to eat and in plain sight. You don't want to feel deprived and you don't want your children to feel that way, either.

Race around the Outer Aisles of the Grocery Store After you know what items you want, you can shop just as fast as you did before — maybe faster — since you will spend most of your time in the outer aisles (where the less processed food usually is) instead of getting tied up in the crowded middle aisles (and perhaps tempted). When you must venture into the middle aisles, go without the cart for quick escapes.

When Food Is Not Enough

In theory, eating from a large variety of nourishing foods should furnish all our nutrients, but busy people rarely can eat an optimal diet. Taking nutritional supplements of vitamins and minerals can make a noticeable energy difference for some people, but not because the vitamins or minerals themselves give energy. These supplements work when the vitamin (or mineral) you take is one that is lacking in your diet, and if it is what you need to "round out the team."

The study of supplements is a complex one; what is offered here is intended only to address the questions people most often ask about vitamins, minerals, and energy. The following is not meant to be a recommendation for your vitamin needs, but an indication of how complex and individual those needs are.

Iron Some fatigue can be caused by anemia, which has several forms. Anemia is caused by more reasons than simply a lack of iron, although this is the most common, especially in menstruating women. It's essential that anemia be properly diagnosed and treated by a medical doctor.

Calcium Calcium has been found to have many uses in our bodies. It may play a role in lowering blood pressure and preventing some kinds of cancer. But a major concern, especially for women is calcium's possible link to bone loss.

Both men and women lose bone mass as they age. If this loss of bone is excessive, it's called osteoporosis, which is painful, disfiguring, debilitating and often leads to fractured bones in the elderly. For women this bone loss is most severe during the five or six years following menopause, but begins when women are about thirty.

Although there is little medical agreement as to the exact cause of osteoporosis, this much is generally accepted: The cause of osteoporosis is complex, an interplay of heredity, hormones and a lifetime of nutritional habits. Specific factors that some researchers believe may play a role in hastened bone loss are stress, lack of exercise, fad dieting, fasting, or ingesting too much vitamin A, coffee, (or cola,) protein or fiber.[52]

Calcium seems central to this condition, although its role is not fully defined. Morris Notelovitz, M.D. and Marsha Ware, in *Stand Tall: Every Woman's Guide to Preventing Osteoporosis*, point out that most American women consume only 450 milligrams of calcium each day from their food. The recommended daily allowance for adults is 1000 milligrams. Dr. Notelovitz recommends 1,200 to 1,400 milligrams a day for women near or past menopause. (One eight-ounce glass of skim milk contains approximately 300 mg. of calcium.)

Doctors have not yet agreed upon the exact roles of diet and exercise on bone loss, but they know that simply taking in the calcium is not all that is necessary. In order to be effective, the calcium has to end up in your bones. For this to happen, it appears that exercise is at least as important as supplements. Vigorous exercise that creates a strain on the bones triggers the release of a growth hormone, which in turn stimulates bone formation in people of all ages.[53] Exercise may be the best and perhaps only way to build and keep strong bones. Exercise that works against gravity, like running, fast walking, weight lifting and strenuous yoga are probably better than activities like swimming, in which little strain is put on the bones.

How to know if you are developing osteoporosis? You don't feel it. By the time you can see it, as a dowager's hump or a curved spine, the damage is done. For this reason, it's known as the silent disease, but here's one clue: If you have a pink toothbrush after normal brushing, this may be a sympton of peridontal (gum) disease, which can be an early sign of insufficient calcium. Tell your dentist. Then take action on your own. Osteoporosis and gum disease are so prevalent, especially among women, that it seems to make sense (while we wait for more research and more definite conclusions,) to take precautions: drink milk, take calcium supplements and exercise vigorously.

The B-Complex Vitamins These vitamins have traditionally been associated with energy level because they are intricately involved with the digestive and metabolic processes. The B-complex group is usually found together in the same foods: in the germ and bran of many grains, nuts, beans, peas (the parts that the refining process removes), and in leafy green vegetables and milk. A food rich in one of the B-complex vitamins is likely to be rich in another. They are also related by function, so if you need one, you probably need more than one, which is why it is usually unwise to take these vitamins singly.

Brewer's or nutritional yeast (*not* baking yeast) is a food, not a drug. It provides the B-complex nutrients (including B^{12}) in natural form. However, if you are taking this, there are some facts you should know. The exact vitamin and protein content of nutritional yeast will vary a great deal, according to Rudolph Ballentine, M.D., in his book, *Diet and Nutrition.* For example, a given batch may contain no vitamin B^{12} at all, which could be serious if you are a strict vegetarian and depend on it as your one source of this necessary nutrient. Moreover, Dr. Ballentine cautions that taking large amounts of nutritional yeast can cause trouble, including elevated levels of uric acid. For this reason he recommends taking not more than one or two tablespoons a day.[54]

Vitamin C   Healthy adrenal glands are essential to the feeling of well-being, so vitamin C is of special interest to those seeking to increase their available energy. Among vitamin C's multifunctions is its use in helping the body rebuild the adrenal glands. The recommended daily allowance for vitamin C is 45 milligrams, but you may need more depending upon your life-style. For example, your vitamin C needs are increased by smoking and by living in a polluted environment.

Everyone has heard about the supposed efficacy of taking huge amounts of vitamin C to fight the common cold. While there are indications that this may work, the safety of ingesting massive doses on a regular basis is open to question. Taking such large doses of any vitamin over a long period of time is self-medication and should be supervised by a professional.

I feel it's wiser to get as many nutrients as possible from food. Several servings of fruits and green peppers or leafy vegetables a day should take care of regular vitamin C needs, for example. People with allergies or other reasons to avoid these fresh foods may need another source.

The preceding vitamins are water-soluble, so excesses will be excreted. The fat-soluble vitamins, however, like vitamins A, D, E, and K, can be stored in the body. An excessive amount, therefore, could be toxic. If you spend time outdoors regularly, eat plenty of green vegetables and yogurt, you probably get enough of vitamins

A, D, and K. Many people take supplemental vitamin E because it is necessary for a healthy heart and reproductive organs. This vitamin is removed from grains by the refining process, leaving little or none in most processed food.

Many doctors recognize that few people eat optimally and are recommending some supplementation. Vitamin and mineral needs are very individual so either be extremely well informed about vitamins or work out your needs with a dietitian or nutritionist.

Drinking Your Troubles Away

What do energists drink?

Coffee? The last word on caffeine isn't in yet, but coffee looks worse with every new study. For an energy lift, coffee is a pretender, granting only a short-term "buzz," followed by the need for another cup of coffee. In the long run, the coffee interferes with the production of endorphine, the body's natural pain-killers that can create a natural high and an intense feeling of peace and well-being. In other words, it deprives you of your own, self-generated good feelings.

Coffee is not good for your health, either. A study at Johns Hopkins University suggests that a person who drinks five or more cups of coffee a day is almost three times as likely to develop heart problems as a person who drinks none.[55] A Minnesota study suggests that heavy coffee drinking increases a smoker's chance of getting lung cancer by seven times.[56] The researchers are in disagreement about the safety of one or two cups a day, but doctors recommend avoiding it completely during pregnancy.

I wish it were possible to say the decaffeinated coffee products are safe. However, a chemical used to remove caffeine has been linked to liver and lung cancer in mice and is being investigated by the U.S. Food and Drug Administration.[57] If you don't drink coffee now, don't start. If you do, try to cut down or stop completely.

Artificially Sweetened Beverages? No one knows whether artificial sweeteners are safe, for whom they are safe, when they are safe, and in what amounts.[58] Certainly, they should be avoided (like coffee and cigarettes) during pregnancy.

Fruit Juices? Freshly squeezed fruit juices are wonderful, but even these don't replace the need for the whole fruit on your daily menu. Some fruits juices (pear, apple, grape, and tomato) can be heated and spiced for a satisfying and warming beverage. In the summer they can be added to carbonated water for a cooling refreshment.

Alcohol? Apparently, the jury is still out on this issue. For most people, alcohol in small amounts is not thought to cause disease, but it can't be said to do anything positive for a person's immediate energy level. While some findings have shown that drinking a moderate amount of alcohol has a beneficial, long-term health effect, these results are not conclusive, and an article in the January 1986 *Harvard Medical School Health Letter* casts doubts on the validity of the research.[59] A little wine enhances a fine meal, but alcohol consumption is one of those things that can get out of hand. In large amounts, it is believed to increase a person's susceptibility to many diseases. An article appearing in *The Journal of the American Medical Association* noted that the risk of hemorrhagic stroke more than doubled for light drinkers and nearly tripled for heavy drinkers. The authors of the article concluded that alcohol consumption is related as well to total mortality, liver disease, and certain forms of cancer.[60]

Using large amounts of alcohol can also interfere with relationships and careers. My informal survey of super-achievers concluded that successful and energetic people don't drink much and don't spend much time on other addictive behaviors, either.

Good Old Water!   Most of your body weight is water. You are a most remarkable recycling operation, using your water many times and most efficiently. What you drink and when you drink it have an influence on your energy level. Sometimes you feel fatigued and think you need rest, when what you really need is a drink of water — good old energizing H_2O.

You cannot depend upon your body's thirst signals to tell you to drink water. By the time thirst registers on your consciousness by providing you with a dry mouth, it's too late; your tissues are already suffering slight dehydration. In one study, male athletes were able to continue on a treadmill much longer when their water loss was systematically replaced.[61] So drink water before you exercise instead of waiting until you are thirsty.

Any good idea can be overdone, and this is no exception. Some weight-loss systems urge the drinking of eight to twelve 8-ounce glasses of water a day as part of the diet plan. This can adversely change your body chemistry.[62] It's best to be moderate about this.

Today it cannot be assumed that all water is good to drink. Over seven hundred synthetic organic chemicals have been identified in the U.S. water supply, and about forty of these are either known to cause or are suspected of causing, cancer.[63] Do you know where your water comes from? Do you know where it is stored? Do you know the distance between it and the nearest chemical waste dump?

For those who investigate and find their drinking water unacceptable, one alternative is bottled water. But don't stop your investigation there! Just because water is in a bottle does not mean that it is pure. Find out the source. Good pure water tastes better and fresher than tap water. The good taste alone will encourage you to drink more.

Keeping It Positive

Think of food choices positively. To say "I choose to eat this because I love me" as you attack a bowl of sparkling garden vegetables or a hot, steamy barley soup is a healthier attitude than concentrating on what you are trying to avoid.

Feeling deprived is an energy enemy. If you fill your grocery cart, your refrigerator, and, ultimately, yourself with fresh, well-prepared, health-giving food, you will feel nourished, not deprived. Eating is fun, one of life's great pleasures. Let it be so!

The wonderful thing about our bodies is how they adapt to whatever we do. When we choose good food over a period of time, our bodies begin to prefer it. Why not? It tastes good!

Pamper yourself! Does a mango or a wild mushroom seem too expensive? Relative to what? Next to a pack of cigarettes or a can of diet cola, they're both bargains. Be good to yourself when you make your choices.

Your Nutrition Quiz

- Do you eat breakfast, lunch, and dinner regularly?
- Do you avoid eating at your desk, standing up, while driving, or otherwise on the run?
- Do you drink four glasses of water every day?
- Do you include plenty of natural-grain fiber in your meals?
- Do you purposefully make low-fat menu choices?
- Do you eat produce that is raw and fresh every day?
- Do you avoid fast-food restaurants?
- Are you conscious of the amount of sugar in the food you eat?
- Do you limit your coffee drinking?
- Do you avoid chemical concoctions (like diet soda) of questionable safety?
- Do you look at your food before you eat it?
- Do you bless your food?
- Do you consider your menu choices overall to be wholesome and health-giving?

Study the questions you answered with a "no." Write here what you choose to improve upon.

_____

_____

_____

_____

Step 4. Creating an Energizing Outer Environment

Does your enviroment give you a lift or depress you? Is it biologically health-enhancing? Aesthetically welcoming? Psychically energizing?

Perhaps it's too much to ask that any environment be all of these. But your physical environment is an important factor in health, energy, and longevity. Super-healthy people are not usually affected negatively by their surroundings. But if you are not experiencing optimal well-being, an environment full of stressful irritants can cause petty and nagging aggravations. An allergy, a state of hypersensitivity to certain things in your environment or your food, can rob you of your energy. An allergy often appears when a person is under stress. The irritation of dealing with the allergy compounds the problem by becoming another stressor. Investigating the cause and cure then, is worth the trouble. Keeping a detailed journal of what you eat, how you feel, your emotional state, and other reactions appears to be the most efficient way for most people to conquer allergies.

In the extreme, environmental stress can cause disease and shorten one's life. But it doesn't have to. We have within us a hard-working and vigilant security force against environmental stress — our immune system. Like patrolling guards with police dogs, the white cells circulate in our bloodstream to keep us healthy by recognizing and destroying foreign invaders such as bacteria, viruses, fungi, and cells whose growth pattern has gone awry. The efficiency of the immune system, previously believed to be outside our conscious control is, as new research suggests, influenced by how we feel and how we live as well as outside factors such as pollution.[64]

We have learned much in the last few decades about the influence of toxins in our food and water, the effects of acid rain on lakes and vegetation, and the tragedies caused by leakages from chemical and nuclear waste plants in different parts of the world. The same has happened on a smaller level: We may be allergic to a substance in our clothing. Some people can't wear wool; others must avoid polyester. Even our jewelry may contain substances that cause irritations. Some buildings endanger their occupants with faulty ventilation systems or insulation materials that contain formaldehyde or asbestos.

We have come to realize that even our "safe" environment is not benign. We interact with it constantly in subtle ways that can enhance our health and energy or affect us with mild symptoms or subject us to potentially life-threatening situations. Before we explore the non-tangible environment, let's look at our physical environment.

The Tyranny of Shoes

It's hard to be lively and dazzling when your feet hurt; and three-fourths of all Americans say theirs do. Although most foot problems are hereditary, an ill-fitting or poorly designed shoe can cause plenty of trouble. When you consider what women are expected to wear on their feet, it's no wonder that most foot sufferers are women.[65] Poor shoe choices have caused lots of people lots of pain, attesting that the price of foot-fashion consciousness is high:

- Pain.
- Distortions, deformities, corns, and bunions.
- Walking is limited, which means stimulating activities like sports, jogging and long walks — just a few of the activities that can encourage good health and energetic living — are probably out of the question.
- In the post-pain stage (after years of ignoring the pain), the damage continues to the feet, even though they no longer register sensation. A certain amount of energy goes into this suppression process.
- When bodily pain is suppressed, pleasure is also.

Being pain-free and able to move easily encourages an energetic life. So be good to yourself and your feet:

- Go to a reliable shoe store that prides itself on personal attention and a good fit.
- When trying on shoes, walk around the store in them for a while before making your decision.
- Don't buy shoes when you are in a hurry.
- Don't buy shoes that feel anything but comfortable.
- Seek out brands that you have previously found comfortable. If necessary, get professional help in determining what kind of shoe is best for you.
- Examine your collection of shoes. Discard those that hurt your feet.
- Massage your feet regularly. Rotate the toes.
- Go barefoot whenever you can.
- For serious problems, consult a podiatrist.

The paradox is that the best exercise for feet is walking — the last thing you want to do when your feet hurt. If you must wear high-fashion shoes for your job, buy well-constructed ones and wear them only when you need them — not to and from work — and take them off whenever you can. I love seeing women in business suits and sneakers! This encouraging trend indicates that we are becoming independent of shoe-fashion tyranny.

Indoor Air Pollution

Our aesthetic sense tells us that a room containing plants is more pleasant than one without. What we feel when we walk into the energizing atmosphere of a room full of growing plants may be more than artful decor. It may be that we are suddenly breathing fresher air.

Research at the National Space Technologies Laboratories suggests that some ordinary house plants have the ability to cleanse the air of three potentially dangerous chemicals sometimes found in homes and offices: — carbon monoxide, nitrogen dioxide, and formaldehyde.[66]

Air-cleaning plants can make a useful contribution to your home or office. They're certainly more pleasing to look at than electronic air purifiers! They seem to "eat" pollutants. B. C. Wolverton, the scientist who did these studies, believes that as few as fifteen plants may significantly cleanse the air in the average home.

The plants that do this heavy-duty work are not exotic species but common, easy-to-grow types like the spider plant, the peace lily, the golden pothos, and the Chinese evergreen. Buy one today and breathe easy.

Smoke Pollution

There is no one magic way for everybody to quit smoking. But there are a great many effective ways. If at first you don't succeed, quit and quit again!
                              Brochure, "Clearing the Air"

If you are a smoker, I wish you well in your efforts to become an ex-smoker. I don't have to tell you why. This chapter is addressed to passive smokers — the people who inhale smoker's exhaust.

Smoke-filled rooms used to be thought of as seats of

power. No longer. People concerned with their health, energy, and longevity do not smoke. People concerned with their children's health do not smoke.

Since many people do not smoke, being protected from other people's smoke and the health hazards involved with proximity to smoke has become an issue.[67] Except in a few states, regulations separating smokers and non-smokers tend to be absent or timidly enforced. While smokers are becoming more aware of the discomfort that their habit causes others, many do not seem to want to acknowledge that passive smoke is downright harmful to the non-smoker.

A survey conducted by the National Institute of Environmental Health Sciences concluded that a non-smoker's risk of developing cancer is increased 1.4 times when living with one smoker. The risk goes up to 2.6 times when the non-smoker lives with three or more smokers. Sharing an office with a smoker probably carries the same risks.

People who lived with three or more smokers, reported the British medical journal *Lancet*, developed leukemia at nearly seven times the rate of people who did not live with smokers. The air that the passive smokers breathe, noted the researchers, is richer in certain carcinogenic substances than the air smokers inhale directly. (It contains fifty times the amount of dimethylnitrosamine, for instance.)[68] With awareness of these facts, "passive smoke" doesn't seem at all passive.

Non-smokers have realized that they are the majority (67%) and are asserting their rights under the banner of "Right to Life, Liberty, and Freedom from Smoke." New health regulations are following this new awareness. Minnesota is leading the states in requiring smoke-free places in public buildings.[69] Find out what your rights are and assert them.

If you don't have any legal rights to smoke-free air where you work, you still have choices. You can negotiate with the smokers or ask to have your desk moved to a smoke-free spot. You can buy a fan or air purifer for your desk, which will make a strong statement. You can try to get your company to join those giving monetary bonuses to non-smokers or employees who quit smoking. You can work for changes in the regulations through your state's smokers' rights group.

Leaving the job because of a smoke-filled environment is extreme, but people *have* done it.

Away from the workplace, nothing can stop you from fighting back. Become active in your local or state lobbying effort for clean air laws. You can patronize restaurants and other places that have non-smoking sections. If you must go to a restaurant that doesn't, help raise the public consciousness by asking for a table in a non-smoking section anyway, even if you've asked twenty times before and your requests were ignored. Eventually, the restaurant management will get the message.

What's hard for the non-smoker is to tell friends who haven't stopped smoking that their smoke is irritating. Do it kindly and wish them well in their efforts to stop.

Getting Free

My friend Marilyn had tried to stop smoking many times. She was celebrating her first anniversary free of nicotine the day she invited me to hear about her struggles to become a non-smoker. As she tells her story, her words show her ambivalence about smoking.

"I was very worried about some women in my real estate office who smoke very heavily. That's why I hired the hypnotist. But I was not going to do the hypnosis myself. I was afraid of the whole thing and I wasn't really ready to stop smoking. It's against my religion to use hypnosis. No, it's the people at our church who don't believe in hypnosis. I don't agree with them, but again, I want to please. . ."

When the hypnotist arrived, Marilyn tried to beg off, but her coworkers would not let her. They pressured her until she agreed at least to be present while the hypnotist was there. So it was not with real motivation that she joined the group.

"We stood in a large circle. The hypnotist said that we should interlock the fingers of both our hands. I had thought that I could not be hypnotized because of my not believing in it, but when he said, 'You will not be able to separate your hands until I tell you to,' I thought, *Ha! That's ridiculous!* I tried to get my hands apart, but I couldn't do it. I tried to relax my hands and I could not. When the hypnotist said that we could drop our hands, I could immediately do it. So I knew that I had been hypnotized. I thought to myself, *If this doesn't work, nothing will.*"

On one level it did work. Now Marilyn easily avoided lighting up a cigarette. But Marilyn's habit had been to use the cigarettes to avoid showing anger. If she became irritated with her husband, Wayne, or if she wanted to spend some of her salary in ways he didn't approve, she wouldn't speak up for herself. Instead, she would acquiesce and bury her feelings by lighting a cigarette as fast as she could. On long car trips it became apparent even to Marilyn what she was doing when she noted how desperately she shuffled the contents of her purse to find cigarettes.

"I have always been extremely uncomfortable expressing anger. In my family it was bad manners to express anger. But underneath was a tigress waiting to get loose. There was a lot of energy, a lot of feeling tied up there, wanting to come out. I was using the cigarettes to keep it in, substituting the 'good' feeling that the cigarette gave me for the 'bad' feeling of a conflict.

"When I stopped smoking I had no other way to deal with this anger. I became loud, obnoxious, and horrible. It was either be so depressed that I couldn't function or let the hostility out. I called Wayne names that I cannot repeat. I did everything verbal that I could because it was such a struggle for me. I threw a lot of dishes. In my saner moments I told Wayne, 'Before I throw the antique china, call the hospital, have them take me away, because then you will know that I've totally lost control.'"

At one point her therapist advised her to start smoking again. "She thought that the hypnotist had really unhinged me. It was that drastic, but I refused to give up."

Wayne was supportive. One by one she and Wayne went through their points of conflict. Marilyn feared that their marriage was going to fold, but with the therapist's help, she persisted. She and Wayne resolved conflicts that had been suppressed for their thirty-three years of marriage.

It took eight or nine months before Marilyn began

to feel free. "I sometimes feel that something is missing, but I am not conscious of wanting to reach for a cigarette. I haven't had any feelings of wanting to get a pack of cigarettes in all that time. I think that's the hypnosis."

Marilyn acknowledges that she could not have done it without the therapy as well. "I can't believe it! I'm calm. I sleep less. I have worked through all the garbage. Now I have learned that I have to just sit up and tell myself, 'Go ahead and do it!' I have to realize that I have a right to do some of the things I want to do, spend some of the money I've earned, and just do what I want. I don't have to ask 'Daddy's' permission!

"Every once in a while when I was a smoker I'd have a spell when my heartbeat was so rapid that I thought I couldn't get my breath. I thought, *You're killing yourself, Marilyn. You're going to be dead if you don't stop*. It used to be a very conscious self-destruct strategy. When things were going badly I would think, *Just smoke a lot! It's socially acceptable and you will be dead in no time*.

"You know what helped the most? My coworkers who wouldn't let me cop out. And my neighbors, who said to me, 'We care too much about you to have you die.' Any expression of affection was a great help.

"There hasn't been a single day that I haven't felt a tremendous increase in energy and self-esteem. My son has an expression. 'All my endorphins are flying.' Several times a day I feel this surge, a real physical surge of energy, and I feel it more all the time. That's what it is. 'My endorphins are flying.'"

The following are some suggestions from the National Cancer Institute to do for two weeks in preparation for stopping smoking:

- Make a list of the positive reasons you want to quit smoking and read the list daily.
- Wrap your cigarette pack with paper and rubber bands. Each time you smoke, write down the time of day, what you are doing, how you are feeling, and how important that cigarette is to you on a scale from 1 to 5. Then rewrap the pack.
- Don't carry matches, and keep your cigarettes some distance away.
- Each day, try to smoke fewer cigarettes, eliminating those least or most important (whichever works best).

Don't buy a new pack until you finish the one you're smoking, and *never* buy a new carton. Change brands twice during the week, each time choosing a brand lower in tar and nicotine. Increase your physical activity. Avoid situations you most closely associate with smoking. Find a substitute for cigarettes. Do deep-breathing exercises whenever you get the urge to smoke.[70]

What happens after you quit smoking? Within twelve hours after you have your last cigarette, your body will begin to heal itself. Within a few days, your sense of smell and taste will return. Your smoker's cough will disappear. You digestive system will return to normal. Most important of all, you will feel really alive — clear-headed, full of energy.

Reach out for help. Many groups are available for people who want to end their dependence upon nicotine or who want to be free of other addictions. Call your local hospital to see what's offered in your community. Phone your local chapter of the American Cancer Society, the American Heart Association, or the American Lung Association. They offer materials, courses in quitting smoking, or referrals to groups that help with other addictions. Why not get all the help you can?

Sound Pollution

Noise hurts us. Loud and intrusive sounds invade our homes and workplaces. The sounds of motorcycles without mufflers, air conditioners, other people's music, ringing telephones, roaring airplanes overhead, chainsaws, screeching trains, and subway cars bombard us daily.

And it's not just our ears that are affected. Being in noisy places can make us tired and drain our energy. Noise can make us tense and angry and ruin our sleep.[71] It can break our concentration and increase our blood pressure. Noise can even be a burden in an economic sense if the proximity to it reduces the value of our home.

Researchers have a lot to say about excessive noise levels. In one study noise was the factor that made people unfriendly and unwilling to help strangers who appeared to need directions.[72] Workers who endure constant high-intensity noise complain of nausea, headaches, sexual impotence, mood changes, and anxiety. Children who were asked to complete a puzzle in a noisy environment gave up more easily than children doing the same puzzle in a quiet room. Children who lived near busy airports tended to become discouraged and give up easily on difficult tasks, a syndrome psychologists call "learned helplessness." The California Department of Health Services reports that children in schools located on loud streets score below their socioeconomic counterparts in quiet schools.

Apparently, the stressfulness of noise may even be fatal. The mortality rate of home dwellers near an airport was 20% higher than for those living farther away. In addition, admissions to mental hospitals were 31% higher, and cases of cirrhosis of the liver due to alcohol consumption were 140% higher![73]

Excessive noise is not the optimal natural state for human beings. And though we can feel the pain of loud noise, we cannot shut our ears against it. What we don't feel is the permanent ear damage it can cause. The noise doesn't necessarily have to be that loud; musicians, whether they be part of a symphony or not, can suffer deteriorated hearing as an occupational hazard.

Although people's hearing often deteriorates as they grow older, young people (who had grown up listening to high-decibel music) who were studied by Dr. David M. Lipscomb "had hearing no better than that of men between sixty and sixty-nine. In effect, these young people were entering their working life with retirement-age ears."[74]

These are ways to cope with environmental noise:

- Purchase quiet appliances and furnaces and insulate those that aren't. (Make sure the insulation material is fireproof.)
- Add insulating furnishings (double carpet padding, carpeting on the walls, upholstered indoor shutters, double draperies, etc.)

- Use ear plugs (though this is not always possible — or safe — on the job).
- Play music to cover unwelcome sounds. Don't use stereo headsets for this. Their sound is wonderful, but it's easy to damage your hearing this way without realizing it. (In animal experiments, 65 decibels of sound — about the same as produced by an air conditioner — caused damage to animal's brain stems.)
- Fix or replace fluorescent lights that hum.
- Plant a barrier of trees and shrubs between you and the source of the noise.
- Learn to "tune it out." (See Step 5 on concentration and meditation.)
- Make friends with immediate neighbors so that it is easy to ask them to turn down their volume when necessary.
- Let restaurant managers know when the music is too loud. (If you have to shout, it is.)
- Take action.

Is noise a problem where you live or work? How do you handle it? Is there anything you can to to change the situation?

Light

Light is not benign. It can influence reproductive cycles, sleep times, eating patterns, and activity levels in animals in ways that we do not yet understand. Why, for example, do hamsters kept in fluorescent light show five times as much tooth decay as hamsters kept in broader-spectrum lighting?[75] And why have male turkeys become impotent after being kept exclusively under ordinary cool-white fluorescent bulbs and recovered after being exposed to lighting that simulated sunlight?[76]

The day/night cycle seems to be vital to our species as well, but to what extent is a question still being explored. This much is known:

- Brightness, color, and timing of light produce chemical changes in our bodies. Light directly influences our hormone production, as it does that of animals.
- Our ability to concentrate and how we relate to others are influenced by the light that surrounds us.
- Light is being used as medicine: Jaundiced newborn babies are exposed to fluorescent lights for a time to regain natural color.
- Light regulates our internal clock. Virtually every function in the body is timed to a day/night cycle (including hormone levels, body temperature, kidney function, etc.)[77] Some researchers believe that the quality of light, whether it is natural or fluorescent, changes the way calcium (and presumably other nutrients) is absorbed into our bodies.

The manipulation of light is being investigated as a way of countering jet lag.[78] Dr. Alfred Lewy reported that people flying from west to east can cushion the jolt of jet lag by getting as much light as possible in the morning at their destination. Conversely, people flying from east to west can speed up their period of readjustment by getting bright light in the late afternoon or evening.

For people who are very light- or season-sensitive, spending more time in natural light or going outside into the light at different times of day may be useful. Manipulation of light helps people with seasonal affective depression (SAD). In this disorder the sufferer becomes irritated, sad, socially withdrawn, anxious, and sleepy (and has trouble getting up in the morning) as the days grow shorter in the fall.[79] SAD patients are treated by extending their hours of daylight with sunlight-simulating (full-spectrum) artificial light. Exposing patients to high levels of light during the early morning or in the evening helps, apparently, because day length, or how long the body believes the day length to be, is the important factor in alleviating this disorder.[80]

Although SAD is a relatively rare syndrome, most people notice negative results when working exclusively in artificial light. Windows in offices are valued, not only as status symbols, but because they seem to enhance our ability to work and concentrate. The cold overhead direct lighting found in most offices is almost universally disliked. People report eye fatigue and headaches more often from this kind of lighting than any other. Fluorescent lights and yellowish sodium lights have been shown to be the most difficult for people who do heavy visual work.[81] Parabolic lenses on fluorescent lights improve the visibility for people who work at computers.

Manipulating the light around you, when it is possible, certainly can change your mood. Some studies show that people work at their best when they have some control over the lighting in their workplace.[82] Carleen, a writer who worked at home, was depressed and desperate to move to another house. Finding this economically unfeasible and sensing that lighting was her problem, she installed skylights instead of moving. Not only has her outlook (and her productivity) improved, but she loves her house and no longer wants to move.

A less-expensive solution for Carleen would have been to purchase full-spectrum light bulbs, which simulate daylight. Full-spectrum lighting, unlike regular incandescent or fluorescent bulbs, simulates the full visible and ultraviolet spectrum of natural white light. These are available from a good electrical supply house.

Natural light in the workplace makes people feel better, but light quality is not the only factor. A window also opens to the world and serves to bring the outside in. It helps people to see the weather and the drama that nature offers. We function best when we have a ray of sunshine and at least a glimpse of the natural setting.

Color

Do you have colors you wear when you are depressed, happy, or angry? What color is your favorite dress or shirt? What color is your favorite place in the world? What color is the room that you like the most? What color was the car you once owned that you are still sentimental about? What color was your partner wearing when you realized you were in love?

Some people are aware of certain colors for which they

have an affinity, and they use them to express their individuality or mood. Others seem to live in a monochromatic world. What most people agree upon is that color influences us greatly. My novelist friend decided to turn what she described as a "dark, depressing, claustrophobic 5-by-6-foot brown room" into her studio. She says that as she painted it white it became "light, spacious and energizing." To her amazement it expanded to an inviting nine-by-twelve-foot writing space — which was its actual size all along.

Color, like light, has been shown to affect us greatly and can be used to manipulate our moods. Have you noticed that fine restaurants are decorated in cool, subtle colors? (They want us to relax and stay a long time.) Or that fast-food restaurants are often an uncomfortable orange? (They want us to eat fast and leave.)

Environmental color, like wardrobe choices, can make a personal statement. Color is close to our emotions and our color choices say much about us. The colors we choose may be those that we know complement us or may be colors we were wearing when a special event occurred, even though the event is long forgotten. Sometimes we choose to wear colors that were worn by an admired friend, even though they may do nothing visually for us at all.

Color can directly express our personalities or become a neutral background for our collections. Some people decorate their homes in the same colors they wear, becoming "one with their decorating." Others choose a basic background or a complement so that they stand out dramatically in their own environment. Women have told me that once they figured out which colors were right for them, using the *Color Me Beautiful* four-season system, they felt energized by their wardrobe.[83] They no longer had "low" days simply because they felt the color they were wearing dragged them down. Some women (and men as well) have embraced the color system as an efficient way to organize a wardrobe and a fast way to clean a closet. Order from chaos is always energizing.

Although colors seem to influence us on an unconscious level in a very individual way, there are some colors, like some symbols, that seem to have larger significance. In yoga the colors of the rainbow correspond to the color assigned to each of the *chakras*, the energy centers on the body identified in ancient Eastern philosophy. If you want to express more love in your life, according to this system, you might focus mentally upon blue-green, which is associated with the heart and love energy, and bring it into your life with dress and surroundings. Orange is associated with fire, the belly, the emotions, and change. Yellow is the color identified with the solar plexus, warmth, and aggressive tendencies.

Whether you believe in *chakras* or body energy centers as fact or metaphor or mythology, the color correspondences they represent seem to be linked to universal feelings about color. Since so many dining rooms are blue, for example, it must reach people on a deep level that blue is a restful color, a perfect background for the important function that takes place there. Blue is instinctively chosen for bedrooms for the same reason.

Insomniacs may want to consider a color like pale blue or a warm, cozy and loving color like peach-rose, thought by many to induce sleep. If you are a person who has trouble getting out of bed in the morning, however, these may not be the most energizing colors you can choose.

Follow your instincts. If you are stressed, anxious, and also dislike both blue and green, it would be counter-productive to create a blue or green room for yourself. If you are bored and looking for changes, bring some orange into your life. But don't make any large investments in orange things. When the expected change takes hold, you will be pursuing a new track and may have new color preferences. Let's look at your own color sense.

Color Awareness Quiz

See what color you find the most:

happy and joyous _____	exciting _____
restful _____	sensual _____
sexual _____	reverent _____
spiritual _____	love-attracting _____
love-giving _____	health-giving _____
youthful _____	timeless _____
calming _____	somber _____
serious _____	businesslike _____
intellectual _____	healing _____
energizing _____	cheerful _____
warming _____	cooling _____
work-inducing _____	

Look at the colors you indicated most often and choose

those with corresponding qualities that you want to bring into your life in greater abundance. Circle these.

Now look through your closet. Clothes express our individuality, self-esteem, and mood. What are you wearing today and what does it say about you? Is this what you want it to say? Are you going with or against your feelings? How about the colors in your house?

You are the authority about the relative values of colors in your life. Each color of the rainbow is open to your own interpretation. What is important is to create an environment for yourself that gives you what you need. Unsure of your own preferences? Knowing your inner self better builds confidence in your own taste.

Perhaps your individual preferences go against those of the crowd and send you different signals. Follow your instincts and don't be bound by color rules; after all, you need only to please yourself.

Creating a Home that Energizes and Renews

A building is more than shelter. Space defines us and the world. There are some spaces that just make you feel happy to be in them. New Englanders tend to be drawn to cozy saltboxes with wood-burning stoves. Westerners and other frontier spirits seem to want open spaces from which to reach out over the horizon. Texas houses seem to sprawl like the state itself.

There is no way to measure exactly the impact of spaces upon our lives, except by gut feeling. You either feel good in a place or you don't. Learning to know yourself is letting yourself trust these feelings.

Don't be embarrassed to refuse to rent or buy if you don't feel right in a space, even if it has the correct number of bedrooms, the price is right, and everyone says it's the best deal in town. Apartments and affordable houses may be scarce, but if one leaves you feeling claustrophobic you'll be miserable living there. Rarely are any places beyond the help of a coat of paint and a healthy dose of imagination, but if one doesn't energize you immediately, keep looking.

You may have reasons, although they are not readily apparent, for being uncomfortable in a space. Maybe it reminds you of something in your past. Maybe you are a "sensitive" who picks up vibrations of past tenants who were unhappy or even tragic.

You have a vision of what "home" is to you. The place you are seeking may be in disrepair and have water in the basement, but if you love the space, creating a home there will energize you.

Whether your living space is a log cabin in the north woods, part of a tiny city apartment, or half of a Winnebago camper, let yourself show. Cultivate your imagination. Celebrate your individuality. Bring in things you love and colors that nurture you. Expressing yourself and what you love in your home can be terrifically energizing.

Surrounding yourself with things that you love and that generate good memories can even be health-enhancing. People's bodies respond by measurable drops in blood pressure and galvanic skin response when they remember loved places. Allow rationality to be put aside when you are deciding what it is you really need in order to feel energized. When you discover it, bring it into your environment. An example: Some people are energized by the ocean. While bringing the ocean home would be cumbersome, you could enjoy "essence of ocean" by hanging a photograph or adding an arrangement of sea shells, an aquarium, fish nets, and driftwood, or a mural of a beach scene. You could even play a tape of the surf pounding the shore.

Do you work at home? What do you need in your work space to facilitate your creativity? Some writers keep their favorite books handy. A composer has a tuned and polished piano free of any objects at all except a dozen freshly sharpened pencils. (No one else is allowed to sit at or play this piano.) Another composer commutes from Wisconsin (where he is a professor) to New York City (where he lives) because he finds the city atmosphere more conducive to his work. A well-known screenwriter who needs absolute isolation in which to work checks into a hotel in a city where she knows no one, carefully choosing a hotel with room service and no bar. She unplugs the phone and stays there until the screenplay is finished.

Listening to your idiosyncrasies may be the key to your creative self. If you, like Samuel Johnson, need "a purring cat, an orange peel, and a cup of tea" in order to work, visit the grocery store and the local humane society to get what you need. Surround yourself with the best your circumstances can offer. In the same spirit, challenge yourself by removing all obstacles to your work. If you still resist your work after you have provided yourself with the optimal environment, perhaps it's time for a serious reevaluation of your goals and job preferences.

What if your work space is dark and depressing, with

only one window that faces another building? What if you aren't allowed to apply paint or hang anything on the wall? What if your sunless apartment is rent-controlled, so you think you cannot afford to leave it? The building doesn't even allow cats or birds or goldfish? Your roomate is allergic to plants? Can you find something here to love? Can you make any small change? A terrarium, perhaps, a small jungle-in-a-bottle, can bring nature into an otherwise dreary space.

You can change your circumstances or you can change your mind about them. If your environment is really dismal, search yourself first and your reasons for being here. Assure yourself that you have chosen this temporary situation and that you will not be controlled by these or any circumstances.

Are you pursuing goals that outweigh your physical circumstances? People have previously sacrificed immediate environment for long-term goals. Maybe it's time to decide you love your goals enough to also love your less-than-perfect environment. As radio storyteller Garrison Keillor says, "When you have love, all places are beautiful."[84]

Whatever your circumstances, tune in to them. Don't anesthetize yourself to your environment. The energy that it takes to "not see, not feel" can be used in better ways. "Notice the world, sense it, react to it, change it," as Dr. James Hillman suggests.[85] Join the great minds of the world who have risen above circumstances and soar above yours.

What you cannot change in your environment, you can use as motivation to spur you on. Brilliant things have been accomplished by persons in reduced circumstances. Constraints can even be the impetus for greatness. To turn your circumstances to advantage, let greatness of spirit, if not environment, be yours.

We all have different dreams of what constitutes beauty, comfort, ease. The very concept of "home" is defined in as many ways as there are people. The purpose of this quiz is to become aware of what makes up an energizing environment for you.

Energizing Your Environment

Choose five words or phrases to complete this sentence: "For me, the optimal home environment is ———"

- secure
- exciting
- calm
- warm
- comfortable
- well lit
- full of friendly faces
- quiet
- orderly
- serene
- cluttered
- rustic
- bright and colorful
- plain and stark
- elegant

- well designed
- close to what I love
- efficient and practical
- non-pretentious, like an old shoe
- sentimental and nostalgic
- high-tech
- other

Are you giving yourself the best you can?

Personalizing the Office

A force even stronger than physical circumstances is the emotional energy that people bring into the places they live or work. Compatible emotional energy is really what you and a potential employer are testing for when you go for a job interview. One of the traits that marks an effective manager is the ability to sense and balance subtle emotional energy shifts within the office environment.

Linda Hoeschler, group vice-president of National Computer Systems, Minnetonka, Minnesota, knows that her own work style is intense and demanding. She buffers this by choosing a secretary who, unlike herself, has a very calm personality. "I looked for a nurturing and very caring person. When I am stressed and am starting to act a little frantic, my secretary will say, 'All right, come and have a cup of tea. Just relax for a while.'" Linda suggests that offices would function better if each level in the chain of command were peopled with opposite types, instead of all hard-driving individualists.[86]

David Dovenberg, a regional vice-president of a Prudential investment subsidiary, personalizes the office he manages with a light touch and a sense of humor. "I can be a tough, mean son-of-a-gun when it's appropriate, but I can also find ways to accomplish the same objective sometimes in a lighter vein. The world is too darned serious."[87]

A retirement party at the office brings out the poet in him. The people he works with look forward to the catchy limericks Dave creates to immortalize these occasions. The person being honored often receives as a personal gift something like a pair of red socks. There's no card with the gift — everyone knows who gives gifts like this — and Dave just grins boyishly.

Not a usual business-suit accessory in the image-conscious world of high finance, red socks are one of Dave's special trademarks. When he wears them to the office, something is special about the day because Dave wears them only when he's in a celebrating mood. The anticipation runs high as everyone speculates upon the cause of the day's good news. Will someone be promoted? Was a multimillion-dollar project approved? Dave lets the rumors circulate, enjoying every moment of the suspense. Finally he makes the announcement. "No, there are no promotions today." "No, the deal hasn't been approved yet."

Why the red socks? Part of Dave's charm is his penchant for the unpredictable.

Again the boyish grin. "It's my daughter's birthday."

This kind of management style is uniquely his own and it works for Dave. What is the emotional-energy environment in your workplace? Can you make it better?

PART II

TENDING YOUR INNER ENERGY SOURCE

Inner Exercise

One of my dogs, Rusty, is a friendly, outgoing, and trusting Brittany spaniel. Rusty's world view is that life is full of irresistibly interesting pleasures and that all people are good.

My other dog, Tess, is a fierce-looking guard dog that jumps at every noise. She's so paranoid that she once snarled at her image in a mirror. Both dogs get what they expect. Rusty's world is filled with sunshine and doggie bones, Tess's with sinister shadows. Rusty, I don't need to tell you, has a lot more fun.

We humans also tend to get what we expect. If I expect that getting my feet wet in the rain will cause a cold, it probably will. If I think like a victim, I'm an easy target. If I believe that illness serves some purpose in my life, some illness will find me. If I accept that I'm powerless to change my circumstances, I probably am.

We grow into the likeness of that which we think — this is inevitable. We attract friends and lovers less by how we look (although plenty of attention is paid to that) or by what we have accomplished than by how we think. Henry Ford said, "The man who thinks he can accomplish something and the man who thinks he can't are both right." Inner exercise is based upon this premise: Everything is a thought before it is a thing. Everything is an idea before it is a product, a life change, a job, an opportunity.

We can take control of our future by taking control of our thoughts and by becoming more aware of what is going on in our inner selves. If we believe that we have power and confidently use all the tools available to us, we can be in the driver's seat of our lives. The first step is to be able to relax. This ability is our key to our interior world.

One practical way to facilitate the process of getting to know the inner self is to keep an inner-exercise notebook recording the date, the method, the time spent, and what happened. Goals, inner dialogue, dreams, new insights, and affirmations can be included. Patterns will start to become apparent, increasing your self-awareness. Dating each entry will provide a good record of growth and change.

Step 5.   Relaxation

When we are relaxed our lives run smoother and easier, our emotions seem more at peace. Relaxed, stress-free people have access to more creative ideas, are generally healthier, sleep less, and have more available energy. Researchers have found that relaxation has health benefits beyond relieving stress and mental tension and can actually prevent some diseases. New studies show that knowing how to handle stress through the practice of relaxation improves the flow of blood to the heart, lowers the blood pressure and cholesterol levels, widens the respiratory passages, and helps alleviate chronic pain.[88] Multiple studies have found that regular relaxation can encourage a healthier immune system.[89] Practicing relaxation regularly may be the best way to avoid catching viruses short of isolating yourself from the world. University health staffs know that it's no coincidence that students have more colds during exam week, when stress is at its highest.[90]

When we are feeling stressed and most need to relax is when relaxation is most elusive. At these moments it's helpful to remember that we still have choices: We can respond to stress by drinking, swearing, or grousing at our coworkers and people we love; or we can relax.

The relaxation activities that work these health advantages are not ordinary ones like catnapping, gardening, or watching TV. Effective relaxation is a specific skill that can be learned. Knowing how to relax at will is more likely to save your life than almost any other skill, except perhaps swimming. The problem most people face is that they don't practice relaxation techniques until they are already severely stressed. That's like trying to learn to swim as the ship is going down.

Once the process of going into a relaxed state becomes a habit, you can do it with a gesture, a word, by assuming a certain body pose or simply with a thought that you have conditioned yourself to accept as the "key" to your relaxation.

Basic Relaxation

Take the phone off the hook. Set a timer for ten minutes. Make yourself comfortable. Lying on the floor is great (not on your bed or on a sofa, where you are likely to go to sleep.) Or you can sit in a straight-back chair if the floor is out of the question.

On the floor you can assume what the yogis call the

"Sponge Posture." Your feet are 18 or more inches apart. If this isn't comfortable, draw your knees up with your feet flat on the floor. Put your hands away from your body, palms up in a "receptive" gesture. Let the floor completely support your weight. If you are sitting in a chair, your feet should be flat on the floor and your hands on your lap, palms up.

Close your eyes. Concentrate on the inside or yourself. Observe the rhythm of your breathing as the air passes through your nostrils, your throat, reacting with the movement of your chest. Breathe in (two . . . three . . . four). Breathe out (two . . . three . . . four . . . etc.). Don't try to change the breathing. Just observe and count.

Be aware that each time you breathe out with the intention of becoming relaxed, you actually do become more relaxed. Let the feeling of relaxation flow over you with each exhalation. Expect it and it will happen.

If your thoughts wander, let them go and bring your attention back to your breathing. When the timer rings, return to the outside world slowly. Now, don't you feel great?

More Relaxation

It seems paradoxical, but one way to become more proficient at relaxation is to be good at tension. Being able to tense muscles at will leads to the ability to let them go at will.

Tension Practice Assume the Sponge Posture and observe your breathing as you did in the previous exercise.

Now clench and tighten your right fist. Make it tighter. Feel your whole arm become tense and tight. Stay with it. Let it become so tense that the arm rises off the floor with the tension. Make it tighter as you count back from ten to zero. Release the tense fist and feel the relaxation flow through the arm. Now do the same with the other arm. Then the right foot and the left.

Enjoy the wonderful feeling of relaxation that you have created. Come back to your outside self slowly, bringing the good feelings of relaxation with you.

Progressive Relaxation (You may want to make a tape of yourself reading this very slowly.) Assume the Sponge Posture. Close your eyes. Breathe normally and easily. Observe your breath for a few cycles. Each time you breathe out with the intention of relaxing, you do become more relaxed.

Let your eyelids be heavy. Let your cheeks be relaxed. Let your jaw be loose. Let your scalp be relaxed. Let the back of your neck be loose and long against the floor. Let your shoulders be heavy. Let your shoulders sink into the floor. Allow the floor to hold all of your weight. Let your elbows be loose. Let your hands be light and warm.

Slowly now. Take your attention back from your hands . . . to your elbows . . . to your shoulders. Check again that your shoulders are relaxed and heavy and supported totally by the floor . . .

Move your attention to your chest and observe how the chest rises and falls with your breathing. Relax and let the breath breathe you. Each breath that you exhale makes you more relaxed. Allow your chest, abdomen, and pelvic area to relax. Let your hips be heavy and sink into the floor. Let your thighs go. Let your knees relax, along with the lower parts of your legs. Now let your feet float, as though they were very light. You are now totally relaxed. Enjoy this wonderful feeling of being relaxed all over. Give yourself several minutes here to enjoy the feeling.

Begin slowly to come back to the outside world by moving your fingers and toes, and by rolling onto your left side before you get up. Before you open your eyes, give yourself a positive suggestion, something that you want to be, have, or do. See yourself as though this was already an accomplished fact. Make a mental image of yourself enjoying this. Be very detailed and specific in your observations.

(If you want to relax further, you can reverse the process by starting at your toes and ending on your forehead, at the place between your eyebrows, the place yogis call the "Third Eye.")

Before you open your eyes, tell yourself: "When I open my eyes, I will feel relaxed, alert, and energetic. I will feel wonderful." And you will. Turn off the tape.

The next step after mastering relaxation is to become more observant of the quality of your breathing. Progressive relaxation with attention given to keeping the breath even, smooth, connected, and sustained can ease fatigue during a busy day.

Once relaxation is mastered, many new techniques are open to you, among them concentration, meditation, affirmations, and visualization. All these are useful as life-enhancing skills that give access to your intuitive self, your inner wisdom. As you allow your unconscious to become conscious, you can go to this source for advice and counsel. You are, after all, your own best guru.

The Energy of Undivided Attention

For the almost twenty years that I have known David Buran, M.D., I have noticed that he seems to concentrate fully on whatever he is doing at any given moment. When we converse, I know he is really listening. When he is making music or playing tennis or discussing art, he is *totally* involved. I have watched David, an otolaryngolist and head and neck surgeon who specializes in treating problems that afflict singers and actors, give his attention to a patient with the same intensity. I asked David how he manages to bring that intensity to each role.

"Commitment," David said. "If I am committed to doing something, I have decided that is what I want to do with that moment or that hour of time. Once I have made the commitment, it is easy to set aside the time, to concentrate on that area for that period of time, even if it just for a few moments.

"I think enjoying is a prerequisite. If I am enjoying I can concentrate upon a subject. That means clearing my mind, being able to do one thing at a time, believing that I will have the energy to get everything done.

"In recent years I have expanded my ability to concentrate so that I can do this most anyplace — my office, with my feet on my desk, or in a noisy train station in South America. I find my place, settle in, and am at peace with that place, even though there may a lot going on around me. I do not want to feel, *It is now time, I must concentrate. I should concentrate.* I want to sit down in a relaxed fashion and have it happen because I am prepared and because I know it will happen."

The ability to be relaxed and yet concentrate fully upon only one subject and think only one thought at a time is a common characteristic of extremely effective people, people who consistently perform at their peak. Such states, new research shows, are accompanied by mental efficiency that feels effortless and enjoyable. Some researchers call these "flow states" — times when the task takes full mental absorption and time seems to fly by unnoticed.

Researchers have found that people concentrate best when there is an optimal amount of pressure, somewhere between too little, when they become bored, and too much for them to handle, when they become anxious.[91]

Noting the relationship between a relaxed state of mind and ease of concentration, David says his relaxed and natural approach to his inner exercise is the result of dropping "shoulds," along with unnecessary guilt and anxiety, from his life. "Having experienced some success and being able to feel better about my personhood have helped me to be able to focus. I no longer have to take on jobs I don't care for to prove things to others or to myself. I think that I'm beyond having to prove to myself or anyone else. I can do what I want to do. I don't have to act any certain way. I don't believe that I am as tied to approval by other people. It's very freeing and allows me to concentrate on what I want to do."

David expands his definition of concentration to include inner exercise that others might term "visualization" or "meditation." David's level of concentration, with feelings of invigoration and relaxed alertness, is like meditation, the essence of which is to focus the attention very completely on one thing.

David's explanation illustrates the relationship of inner and outer work. The dropped "shoulds" and the successes experienced in his outside life helped him to reach a deeper source in his inner life. Concentrating better inside helped him to function better in his daily life and brought him more successes.

Learning to concentrate intensely and thoroughly on one subject at a time increases our effectiveness in the world. And the better we are at concentrating, the easier it is to access our interior world, whether we are visualizing, affirming, or doing Eastern meditation. Like a grand circle, it's all related.

WordSpinning

We are creatures of words, and we have within us important ideas that are often on the tip of the tongue or hidden inside the pen, but not easily accessible to us. Word-Spinning frees up information stored in the right side of your brain and lets it bubble up into your consciousness. It's a way to sweep out the corners of your mind, to remember dreams or real events, and to learn what's really going on inside yourself. If something is bothering you, you can use WordSpinning to search the subject out before you take action.

WordSpinning is a way to activate the more creative

and intuitive aspects of your thinking and to make connections that previously may have gone unnoticed. As a preparation for writing a letter, speech, or report, WordSpinning helps clarify and develop fuzzy half-thoughts into usable ideas, finding connections, like metaphors and illustrations, to enrich your writing.[92]

As a preparation to concentration or meditation, or even before a good night's sleep, WordSpinning is an efficient way to clear your mind. There are no rules for WordSpinning, except to write down everything that comes to mind — no matter how far off the track it may seem — without judgment or criticism, and to avoid lines of words, like linear sentences and vertical columns. The theory here is that the right brain likes circles more than lines and columns. I think of this as a round outline that helps me collect, develop, and connect my thoughts.

Let's suppose that you have a decision to make. You are at a juncture in deciding between several alternatives. In order to learn what you really want, follow these prescribed steps:

1. Relax, using one of the techniques explained earlier
2. Answer one of the following items:
   - "I want . . ."
   - "What I really want is . . ."
   - "What I want most and am willing to commit myself to is . . ."
   - "What I want most to be free of is . . ."
3. Write the word or phrase that completes your sentence in the *Middle* of a large piece of paper. *Do not write it at the top!*

4. Draw a circle around the phrase.

5. Immediately write the next word or phrase that pops into your head beside, under, or over your first phrase. Connect the phrases with a line. Keep your pen moving in circles, darkening the previous circle until a new word comes.

6. Add the next word that spontaneously occurs to you. Continue to the edge of the page until you run out of words or space.

7. Return to your first phrase in the middle and "spin" in another direction. You may find another word along the way that precipitates its own "spin-off." The pattern on the page is not important. What *is* important is to keep the pen moving and to allow yourself to be spontaneous as you fill the space with words inside circles.

8. Continue writing words or retracing circles until the page is full or ten minutes have passed.

9. Assess what you have written by writing a short paragraph in your inner exercise notebook that begins, "What I learned was . . ." or "I was surprised to find that . . ." or "What I really want is . . ."

Did the exercise give you any new insights? If not, try again on a different day. You can WordSpin on any word or phrase. The preceding steps are particularly useful for clarifying your goals. You may have learned, for instance, that you are not putting your time and energy focus behind what you really want. Lighting a fire under your energy source may be facilitated by focusing your energy in the direction of your goals. Women particularly tend to serve others' needs before their own and to hold a secret goal while putting time and effort into something else. This is a sure cause of fatigue.

Visualization

Visualization, the making of imaginary images, is not mysterious or weird when you consider that you do it easily and naturally. What is daydreaming if not visualizing images? What is planning if not seeing the anticipated scene in your mind? Visualizing a situation positively before living it — whether it is a sport, a social situation, a job interview — helps good things come true. Visualizing the worst that can happen — a surprisingly common habit — probably encourages undesirable results. What is worry, for example, if not a negative visualization of the future? These negative worry images, if vivid enough, can sometimes act to become self-fulfilling prophecies.

The late John Boyle, originator of the Omega Seminars, used this illustration: "If you are so worried about hitting a tree that you watch all the trees very carefully, you will certainly hit a tree. On the other hand, if you ignore the trees, and don't even look at them, but keep your eyes glued to the road, you will safely pass the trees and continue toward your way."[93]

There are different ways to approach mental image-making: Passive Visualization, and Active Visualization.

Thoughts that seem to come spontaneously from inside are sometimes called Imaging or Passive Visualization.

Passive visualization is like daydreaming. The thoughts flow in without your consciously willing them, much as birds fly in and out of your field of vision when you are outdoors. They fly in, through, and away. All you need to do is observe.

In Active Visualization, you make a deliberate choice of a goal, then concentrate upon the image of yourself realizing this goal. Athletes use active visualization to help themselves achieve new skills and set new records. This kind of mental image-making has been discovered to be a great learning tool, both in business and in education. We can benefit from positive, deliberate, and purposeful mental image-making in our personal lives.

Active Affirmation is doing the same with words instead of images, what some might call "talking to yourself." The word *affirmation* means "affirming or asserting something as true or real." When you are affirming, you are saying what you want to happen as though it already is happening. Like visualization, it's an effective way to make changes intentionally in your life. Everyone seems to have a running dialogue with a "friend" on the inside anyway, so you may as well make sure that it's a good friend, and that the words represent what you really want to happen.

While it may not be possible for us to have *everything* we visualize or affirm ("I see myself on my own yacht"), the first step to any achievement is to visualize what we want to happen. We don't get degrees, jobs, or homes we want — any of our goals — without first making at least a general image of the desired result. Active affirmation or visualization is honing this natural skill for more efficient use. This is not hocus-pocus but mental preparation. A rational, non-metaphysical explanation is that holding the mental image focuses our attention toward the desired result. This prepares us to recognize opportunities and act when these opportunities present themselves.

A constant dialogue goes on in our heads. It's normal, and there's no way to turn it off. These thoughts, even those that are negative and self-defeating, seem to be charged with their own energy. Thoughts like "Nobody likes me" and "If I don't get this promotion I'm a failure," if allowed to rule us, can become self-fulfilling prophecies.

When you converse with yourself or when you give yourself a specific mental image, you are programming your "bio-computer" to perform in a certain way. One of the ways in which your inner self differs from a computer is that it receives visualizations as well as verbal commands. Yet, like a computer that acts only upon the quality of information it is fed, your inner self reacts to the kind of messages you give it.

This powerful mechanism works all the time, so you may as well take control of it. Your receptive mind is your best friend and can work with you or against you. Consider what happens when you give yourself a negative message: "You dummy! Did you make that same mistake *again*?" Or: "I'm terrible at math." Or: "I'm terrified of public speaking." When the inner self starts to believe all this negativity, it acts as though it were so. What a waste of energy to work against ourselves in this way! Since we tend to get what we hold in our minds, better to call up the images of success. You don't need an inner self who is intent upon scoring goals only for the opposing team!

Thought Replacements

Everyone has a full list of things that could have been done better. Old resentments, omissions, and thoughtless acts (our own and those of others) can crop up to bother us, like gremlins making mischief. If you let your mind dwell upon them, these thoughts just get bigger and bigger and produce what I call "the snowball effect."

The most popular gremlin seems to be self-criticism. It's inhibiting and energy-draining, a habit born of acquiescing to the criticism of others or of continually expecting too much of oneself. Although the "facts" this gremlin tells us may be true, the criticism gremlin lies. All these "facts" are useless history and have nothing to do with your situation today or your worth as a human being.

You don't have to listen to the criticism gremlin. Whenever you catch yourself criticizing yourself, substitute a purposefully chosen positive affirmation. For example, if your gremlin says, "You're a terrible driver," counter with: "I enjoy being a safe and confident driver." If your gremlin says, "You can't write," replace it with: "I enjoy and am successful at communicating through writing," or, "I can write if I choose to." Some people use a gesture as well, like moving the arm as though to close a door on the gremlin, or as a windshield wiper "cleaning the negative thought away."

If yours is a particularly vicious gremlin who tells you things like "Nobody likes you," you can fight back with thought replacements. If your gremlin is very persistent, you may need to be more aggressive and do formal affirmation sessions to dislodge the culprit and work on your self-esteem as well. These are covered in later sections.

Luckily, the snowball effect is just as powerful when it works in reverse: The kind of energy it takes to be in a bad mood or think poorly of yourself can be turned around if you shift gears and replace the negative thoughts with better ones. If you give a positive thought the same intensity you gave to the gremlin's monologue, its influence in your life will also snowball. Choose a specific thought replacement from those offered at the ends of the sections in this book or one of the general statements in the following list:

- I am kind and lovable.
- I trust myself.
- I enjoy being completely confident in all situations.
- I deserve the best that life has to offer.
- I love life.

Don't lose energy because of your mind's random and mischievous memory bank. Every time a negative, self-destructive thought pops up, use it as a reminder to say or think your chosen positive statement. After a while, the more positive thought will appear automatically.

Formal Affirmations

You don't have to wait for a negative thought to pop up in order to give yourself a better one. Practicing formal affirmations once or twice daily for at least ten minutes in a relaxed and receptive mood is an effective way to make important changes in your life.

After you are relaxed (using one of the methods in this book), read positive phrases several times out loud. You could also write them down, twenty times each. The easiest way is to play a tape of yourself reading your affirmations along with relaxation instructions. (You can buy prerecorded affirmation tapes, but why listen to someone else's voice? Unless hearing your own voice makes you uncomfortable, record your own.)

You may make an affirmation for any area in your life in which you seek changes. The most powerful place to institute change is in the area of self-esteem and well-being. When your self-esteem rises, your life changes for the better. When you are feeling healthier, you like yourself better. So I propose that you focus first on self-esteem and well-being. Self-esteem affirmations are the fast track toward achieving a strong energy-generating center. The following are examples of affirmations that enhance self-esteem. You never can get too much of these![94]

- I love and accept myself just as I am. (Or: I love myself unconditionally.)
- It's easy for me to be relaxed and centered.
- I am free. (Or: I am free to live up to my own expectations and I release others from having to live up to mine. Or: I am free from guilt and resentments.)
- My energy level is harmonious to my needs.

- Every day I am becoming healthier in mind and body.
- I trust myself.

An affirmation or visualization is not forever. You may change it whenever the goal is accomplished or has been replaced with another. If you find that your interests have led you to seek another goal, let this one go. Do this whenever you have a major change. It is not useful to affirm something that is already accomplished.

You can create your own customized list of affirmations by using those you find at the ends of the sections in this book. Use your Inner Exercise notebook to record new affirmations when they become appropriate and, if you wish, results of old ones. First copy in the basic self-esteem and well-being affirmations. As you continue reading this book, copy into your notebook other affirmations or thought replacements that you find particularly appropriate. Keeping your list handy makes it easier to regularly practice your inner exercise. Again, if you date each entry, your notebook can be your personal record of growth.

Letting Go of the Present

"I can't say those things," I said when I was first introduced to affirmations. "It's like lying to myself."

Is your mind resisting the idea of affirmations? Mine resisted wildly. I was bothered by the idea of stating something that I didn't see as a true, accurate, and absolute fact.

I was stuck in certain habits and attitudes. By questioning the ethics of affirmations, I was excusing myself from the risk of having to change. By clinging to the truth of the present, I was also denying that what I wanted in the future was a possibility. With this attitude, I was like a boulder in my own path for change. I moved the boulder by doing affirmations. Then I started to believe in my own possibilities.

What was holding me back was the fictional nature of affirmations. It didn't seem right to say things that were not yet true, even though I was saying them only to myself.

And yet this is a way to cope with a less-than-perfect situation. Concentration-camp survivors tell of keeping themselves going by sharing visualizations of how good life would be after their ordeal was over.

Maybe you feel resistance to the idea of affirmations because you aren't ready for change. If so, accept this for now. Where you are is the right place for you to be. With each new day you have the chance to choose again for something different.

Some individuals resist affirmations because they fear they're not worthy; it is a type of fear that "good cannot happen to me unless bad happens to someone else." Life doesn't have to be a win/lose situation. It can just as well be win/win. Are you happy for your friends when something good happens to them? Are they happy for you? Good. Make your friends happy by allowing good things into your life and by expecting that good coming to you will be good for others as well. If this is one of your issues, you can end your session with these words: "This, or something better, is in store for me, reflecting my desire to receive blessings that are for the highest good of all." Write this down in your notebook, too.

You don't know what you want to affirm? Go back to the section on WordSpinning, and spin the phrase to fill in the blanks after "I want . . ." or "What I really want to happen is . . ." Then write the strongest, most positive results in your notebook as though they have already happened.

Wording Your Affirmations

To change a desire into an affirmation, replace the words "I want . . ." or "I wish ..." with "I enjoy being . . ." or "I enjoy having . . ." Make it a clearly positive, present-tense statement, and be as concise as possible.

You can minimize your potential by being too specific. Beware of repetitions such as "I want my boss's job." This would be more productively affirmed as "I love my interesting, challenging, and financially rewarding career." (Why limit yourself to your boss's job? There may be something much better out there for you — like your boss's boss's job!)

"I want my old lover back" is similarly limiting. Better is one of the following: "I enjoy attracting loving, happy relationships into my life," or, "The more I love myself, the more I love others."

The affirmations work best when they are accurate, detailed, positive, and in the present tense. To pump more energy into your affirmations, visualize the situation in your mind's eye at the same time, or mentally review the feeling you expect to get from the realization of the thought.

Incorporate the word *enjoy* into your phrasing whenever you can. It's also helpful to feel or remember enjoyable instances while you are practicing. It won't do much good to gain your heart's desire if you are not going to enjoy it, so you may as well program the enjoyment in with the message. Your inner self is more receptive to enjoyable messages. You will go further with "I enjoy being free of cigarettes," (or simply "I am free") than "I'm not going to allow myself to smoke anymore."

"I want my pain to go away" becomes more powerful when revised to "I enjoy a comfortable, happy life." It's usually better not to mention pain or the name of a disease or a negative condition in your affirmation. Giving a disease a name gives it power it doesn't deserve. Saying "I am free" is enough. Your body knows from what it wants to be free.

You want positive changes, so give yourself *only* positive messages. Always use positive words, and avoid negative ones, such as *no*, or *don't*, or *not*. Most sentences containing negative words can be rephrased in a more positive way. Just listen to a life-insurance salesperson give a pitch!

Choose wording with which you feel very comfortable. If you cannot feel good about the affirmation, change it, but be careful the rewording doesn't give it a different meaning. If "I love and accept myself just as I am" is difficult, try something more modest for a while, such as "I love myself more every day." Proceed boldly but thoughtfully. Remember, if it's not a little bit fictional, it's not a useful tool for change.

Some people have received wonderful results using visualization and affirmation for wealth, objects, and career positions. I think this is all right to do, although I'm more comfortable with affirming for things that are intangible, like job satisfaction, good relationships, happy families, good health, and energy. I caution you to make sure that you really want whatever you visualize or affirm for. And always add the phrase about achieving only what is "for the highest good of all."

More detailed and sophisticated affirmation/visualization skills can be learned from various seminars like Omega.

R_X: A Fighting Spirit

> I was not ready to die! I was not even going to accept the idea that I was going to die! Life is just too wonderful.
>
> — Penny Jacobs,
> February 1985

How powerful are affirmation and visualization? Can these techniques actually influence our health and well-being? Is attitude important in healing illness? The debate about this rages in medical and psychological circles. One who believes that attitude counts is Penny Jacobs. Energetic Penny is one of medicine's "exceptions." She is alive and well eleven years after she was told she had less than two years to live.[95]

In 1975, Penny, her husband, Sol, my husband, and I went to a French film titled *Cleo from Five to Seven*.

The story follows a woman's inner journey for two hours (five to seven o'clock, covering the time from when she learns that she may have cancer until the suspicion is confirmed). After the movie, Penny said to us, "That's exactly what is happening to me. My abdomen is growing larger for no reason. My pants don't fit. I know that I have cancer."

Although pants not fitting is not a usual cancer symptom, an enlarging abdomen on a slim frame like Penny's (when she knew she was not pregnant) was cause for concern. We urged her to go to her doctor. Penny's worst suspicions were confirmed. The reason her clothes no longer fit was that she had an ovarian tumor the size of a grapefruit plus other malignancies. She underwent extensive surgery, but inoperable cancer remained. Thirty radiation treatments and chemotherapy followed. The doctors told her that two years was the longest she could expect to live.

A cooperative but strong-willed patient, Penny was a fighter and a lover of life. A grade-school teacher, a mother of four, a photographer, a naturalist, a political activist, a skier, Penny was always on the move. Naturally outgoing and energetic, she was determined to mobilize every one of her many resources for her own recovery. Throughout her ordeal, she continued to do what she loved: walking, bicycling, swimming, canoeing — anything that could be done outdoors in Minnesota. The outdoors, says Penny, is her "religion".

"Freeing myself to preserve my energy is a kind of mental attitude I believe in. 'No matter what happens,' I say, 'I'm not going to let this thing drain me of my energy.' Energy is something that I want to keep in balance.

I don't allow myself to lose that, no matter what happens. I made a deep decision about my energy that is strong like a religious belief. Nothing interferes with my energy, and that went for my cancer as well."

In the course of the illness, Penny really had to struggle to keep up her energy. "With no energy and a very poor prognosis, I had to find new ways to keep myself going. I started to write. I wrote poems, funny things, very serious things. I just wrote whatever my feelings dictated which was extemely therapeutic. I ended up writing a whole book about my experiences. I feel like I am the luckiest person in the world."

Research has confirmed that patients like Penny, who saw themselves as active, strong, and believed that they could fight their disease, seemed to survive longer than those who reacted to their disease passively as victims.[96]

Dr. Carl Simonton and psychologist Stephanie Mathews-Simonton developed a visualization therapy for cancer patients to encourage this fighting attitude. This was to be used along with, not instead of, traditional cancer therapy. This system is based upon the premise that the patient's self-image is an important element in the prognosis of the disease and attempts to change the patient's attitude to one of strength.[97] Patients were taught to relax and to visualize their own cancer-fighting cells in concrete images — strong, ferocious animals, wolves, lions, bears, attacking cancer cells.

Penny Jacobs (who was not a Simonton patient) used a variation of the Simonton system in her own visual-izations. Since she believed in her innate energy and had a good mental picture of it, she visualized her energy as a flame that "burned up the cancer." She practiced this routinely as she underwent radiation and chemotherapy. She held this visualization during her rest periods following the therapy sessions and during her long, brisk walks.

Did Penny's mental attitude play a role in her survival? Did her visualizations strengthen her immune system? Does the Simonton system work? Many think so. This concept has been used by many patients successfully to bolster their immune system while they received standard cancer treatment.

Every virus, microbe, or foreign particle that invades our bodies triggers some kind of immune response. Stress also seems to play a role in our immunity to disease though it is not the nature of the stress itself, but of our reaction to it that seems to make the difference. Psychologist Sandra Levy studied personality factors as related to natural killer (NK) cell activity and the spread of cancer to the lymph nodes in women treated for breast cancer. Women who maintained a passive attitude, accepting and adjusting to the disease, showed lower NK-cell activity than those who responded with anger.[98]

Those like Penny Jacobs — feisty people who want to play an active part in their own treatment — seem to have a better chance of recovering than those who passively accept the finality of the disease. Those who believe that their bodies can heal themselves, who want and plan on their recovery and are willing to fight for it, using all means possible, may actually have a better chance of doing just that. Having hope or faith in their ability to heal themselves or having faith in a higher power is helpful, perhaps because this kind of attitude can help combat debilitating depression.

How these responses and our emotions, thoughts, and stresses are connected remains to be explored. New evidence of the mind-body link is becoming available as researchers become increasingly interested in this field. In recent studies at Harvard, students who were identified as being easily engrossed in thoughts and images were trained in muscle relaxation and then asked to visualize certain specific images. Relaxation alone increased defenses against upper respiratory infections. By adding imagery, the effect was even stronger.[99]

Enhancing our natural ability to heal ourselves by changing our attitudes and beliefs has been interpreted by some as a way to "blame the patient for being ill." This is not my intention in presenting this material. I'm not saying that you can catch a cold or get cancer just because you're feeling depressed or tense or hostile, but emotions and stress clearly contribute to the onset and course of the disease. We know how to counteract this. We don't expect to do the impossible. But we can sometimes do the yet unexplained.

While medicine is waiting for solid documentation on the validity of this approach, we can learn to use these techniques and see for ourselves. *This is not recommended as a substitute for medical treatment or sensible action.* (You cannot expect affirmations to lower your serum cholesterol level, for example, unless you are also following your physician's instructions for diet and exercise.)

So why not use all the tools available to us for health and energy? I never heard of anyone being hurt by adding a strong and optimistic attitude or a vision of well-being to whatever professional treatment is being offered.

Ups and downs, varying degrees of well-being, are

human and a natural part of living. None of us needs to believe we cause our own illness. Whatever your state of health, look forward, not back. Look up, not down. Love yourself for what you are while you hold a clear image of what you want to become next.

The Process of Eastern Meditation

> Listen to the silence inside you.
> — Mother Theresa

Both Eastern and Western methods for inner exercise are beneficial. There is no reason not to master and use both techniques.

Active affirmation and visualization are practices of choosing your thoughts or "programming" your mind as though it were a computer. These two techniques have been called American meditation because they often produce quick and easy results. American meditation differs from Eastern meditation methods like TM (transcendental meditation), in which the point of meditating is to free the mind from the intrusion of thoughts. In spite of its introspective nature, Eastern meditation is not a negation of the outside world. More accurately, it builds a bridge between the external and internal self. With Eastern meditation, you can improve your relaxation skills, learn to "tune up," and really get in touch with your inside self, which helps you learn to trust yourself and see things more clearly. Some people call it "clearing the air between their ears." In addition to finding more creative and intuitive powers, many meditators have come in closer contact with the natural world and are attuned more easily to the feelings of others. Meditation can be either a secular or religious experience, depending upon what is desired and expected. Best of all, meditation helps you learn to trust yourself.

Meditation is not an end in itself; as a quest toward clarity and inner understanding, it is a search with many side benefits. It's a way to meet and objectively clarify your relationship to the person you are. It's a way to learn your real hopes and aspirations, and identify who you are in relation to the outside world. Some, like Mother Theresa, refer to listening to the "silence" inside or of getting to know the higher self by shutting out the sounds and senses of the physical world.

Paradoxically, it is also the practice of letting go — of resentments, distractions, bad memories — by becoming like an empty vessel. The emptiness makes room for new perspectives. Eastern meditation can bring many temporary physiological changes, including reduced tension and anxiety. To reduce these stresses can mean a very real and easily available energy source. It's a natural process, like prayer or mulling over a problem. It helps one take control of the inner world.

Some believe that the current interest in meditation is a sign of a new evolutionary leap for mankind, a step toward bridging the alienation we have toward our world and one another. The idea is that by changing our thinking as individuals, we can be part of a "global affirmation" toward a peaceful future. Meditation has been called "the Earth's move for self-preservation."[100]

Pope John Paul II acknowledged the global value of

Eastern philosophies on his 1986 visit to India when he said, "India's greatest contribution to the world can be to offer it a spiritual vision of man. And the world does well to attend willingly to this ancient wisdom and in it to find enrichment of human living."[101]

Choosing Your Inner Exercise Style

There are many types of inner exercise from which to choose: prayer; "mulling" and interior silence of the Christian tradition; saying the rosary of Roman Catholicism; silence, as practiced by the Society of Friends; the "stocktaking" of Judaism; Raja Yoga as practiced by the Hindus; Za-Sen or "just sitting" as practiced in Buddhist traditions. Chanting is common to many traditions. And of course, there is American meditation.

Eastern meditation provides a way of quieting yourself, of being open to your subconscious voice, of going inside to find your answers. You quiet yourself by thinking of only one thing at a time. The tool with which to do this is the *mantra*.

The mantra is a word or phrase that is repeated silently or chanted aloud. Chanting aloud is particularly powerful, because you are both originating the sound energy and receiving it when you hear yourself. In the same way, joining your energy with others by chanting with a group can be powerful and energizing.

When initiated into yogic traditions, a swami gives the initiate words upon which to meditate, but it is not necessary to do this before you can begin to meditate. You can just as well choose words from your own religious tradition. Christians might choose something like "Thy will be done," "*Kyrie eleison!*" or "My peace I give unto you." Jews and Christians might be comfortable with the Hebrew phrase meaning peace on earth, "*Shalom chaverim.*" People of many religious traditions could join the Moslems in repeating *ahadum*, or "One," as in "One God."

A mantra doesn't have to have meaning. You can simply breathe in on the word "one" and out on the word "two." These two numbers are repeated. If you want foreign-soundings words, try breathing in on the word "sat" and out on the "nam." Or breathe in on the word "so" and out on the word "hum." Coordinating a mantra with your breathing is another way to make your meditation more effective.

Chanting sustained sounds of "Om" is used in hatha yoga classes because it is denominationally neutral (derived from the same root word as "Amen") and energizing. "Om" is called "mother of all mantras," and "the unity from which all diversity exists."[102]

For mantra meditation, sit with your spinal column straight in a chair or cross-legged on the floor. Be comfortable. Start chanting your chosen phrase aloud, but not loudly. (Stop if you become dizzy or start to hyperventilate.) Keep chanting and do nothing. Think of nothing else. Let the chant fall into a natural rhythm and continue that. Attempt to become aware only of your chanting. This takes some discipline. After a few weeks you'll know if this is the kind of meditation for you.

The object of your concentration can also be visual. It can be a circle that you have drawn on a piece of paper, a colorful mandala, or a religious icon. Some people choose a natural object, a beautiful rock, or a flower. Others light a candle and stare into the flame. Whatever you choose, it serves the purpose of drawing you into yourself. It is a way of signaling yourself to shut out all distraction and concentrate on this point. You are not worshipping the object you use as your focus; you are using it as a key to entering an inner part of yourself.

Buddhist-type meditation is called "one-pointed" or "empty mind." Westerners are often baffled by the whole idea of "empty mind." The following Buddhist story told by the Rev. Robert Corin Morris illustrates this well.

There once was an old peasant who went to the church each day for an hour and sat at the back looking toward the alter, containing the holy bread. He showed no devotional behavior, said no prayers, rattled no beads. Finally, the priest stopped the peasant one day and asked, "What is it you do each day?"

"Nothing," replied the old man. "I just look at God, and God looks at me."[103]

The old man had found the state of mind called "one-pointedness" or "empty mind." Although it is possible to slip into a light meditative state naturally, going beyond this light contemplative state to the stronger experience of "middle way" or "empty mind" meditation takes intention, intense concentration, commitment, and practice. This meditation, its proponents will tell you, is not like anything else. It's not the same as affirming or visualizing. It's not like fantasy or reverie, although these are also altered states. I have not included instructions on this type of meditation because I believe that this deep meditation requires a good teacher.

There is no best way to the inner self, so don't be

afraid to change traditional practices to suit you own needs.[104] The matter is very individual and the best way for you may be more than one method and many teachers. Keep an inner exercise notebook or record your progress on your calendar. Include date, exact time you meditated, how long the session was, and what happened, if anything.

All inner exercise is hard work, but if the system you choose is right for you, it will make you feel better after a month of so. All meditation techniques are best learned from a qualified instructor. So choose your teacher carefully. Steer clear of any who ask: 1. unquestioned obedience; 2. you to be isolated from your friends or family; or 3. that you keep what you learn a secret. Don't continue with a practice if it doesn't feel right. Stop, take a break, try something else. When your energy is flowing freely, when inner exercise is hard work but feels good, then you know that the path is right for you.

Meditation can change people profoundly. Choose your system thoughtfully, keeping in mind your background, personal philosophy, and what would create the best balance in your life.

Inner Confidence/Outer Change

"My energy was so blocked. At that time I was forty years old. My body was in terrible shape. I was smoking three packs of cigarettes a day. I was thirty pounds overweight. I was tired all the time."

It's hard to believe that slim, joyous, and vital Moira, now a successful psychotherapist, is describing herself as she was twenty years ago. Moira has two master's degrees and a successful therapy practice. She conducts workshops, teaches, lectures, and shares her joy and vitality with others. She explains how things used to be.

"I was tired all the time, very drained, very anxious. Because I was a perfectionist, the spontaneity, the playfulness, and all that motherhood at its best can be was stifled. Motherhood was a duty. I knew that I had fun and spontaneity somewhere, but could not find it within me. I wasn't able to express it until I decided, after my children went to school — all four of them — that I was going back to high school. [I had not graduated from high school because I had run off to get married at the age of seventeen.]

"I took a G.E.D. [the High School Equivalency Exam] and started college. I thought what I would do was to get some education and then get a divorce. This was the very early sixties and I was in college with a group of young people. I was in my forties and one of the first mature students to be in college. My husband resented my going back to school terribly, but something inside was telling me that there was more to life than this traditional, stringent environment.

"When I became involved with this younger group of people, I began to feel very young, too. There was a student, a young man, who said to me, 'I would like you to work with me in a psychology program in transcendental meditation.'

"Transcendental meditation! You can imagine how that went over with my very straitlaced and traditional family, but I agreed and became very involved with the TM group. I found that my energy level after meditation was so high, and there was such clarity in my perspective. It totally energized my whole sense of being.

"Once I started enjoying this good feeling, I wanted more of it. I wanted to find more of this energy inside myself that I could release and bring forth. I changed my attitude toward my family and my attitude toward life because I saw that there was another way of being and I was finally giving myself permission to be it.

"After I began meditating, I became involved, because of the Vietnam War, in draft counseling through the college with the Society of Friends. All that was happening resulted in my doing things I didn't believe I was capable of doing when I thought I was just a housewife. Meditation opened me to my life's possibilities!"

Part III

OVERCOMING INNER ENTANGLEMENTS

Step 6.   Turning Anger Around

In this part we will examine ways to get through the most common energy obstacles. All of us have experienced these in some form. Who has not felt some anger, stress, depression, lack of self-esteem, envy, or drive for perfectionism (and its cousin, procrastination) at one time or another? These are normal reactions to difficult situations. When they became abnormal is the time when they persist in keeping you from being the joyous, energetic being you were meant to be.

Anger, like stress, is an umbrella word, that has complex cause-and-effect relationships to other emotional states, as well as to your total health. Many emotions that we define separately are variations, extensions, and cover-ups for anger and fear: guilt, depression, envy, drive for perfectionism, among many. I suggest that you move slowly through this section, doing the exercises when they seem relevant to you.

Anger is probably the first emotion you felt when, as a newborn, you were forced to leave a warm, safe womb to be thrust into a cold and hostile world. You wailed with a fury, punching the air wildly with your tiny fist and feet every time you were hungry, wet, cold, or feeling neglected. It was a fast and effective way to get results.

According to the "fight or flight" theory, you were born knowing this angry behavior. It was part of your survival system, left over from millions of years of service as a hunter-warrior. In those days, if this theory is correct, what made the difference between your becoming a lion's dinner or a local hero was your ability to respond to threat or challenge by becoming physically more able. Your young warrior's body received a sudden spurt of adrenaline and a surge in blood-sugar level, which made you more alert, faster, stronger, and fiercer. (It's not reported what women were doing through all this.)

So here you are, the smart baby, all grown up in a high-tech age with an anachronistic survival system. When you feel that your safety is threatened, your body prepares instinctively for fight or flight. You're ready to fight or turn and run from danger. This response may have served our ancestors well, and it is still useful to us in emergencies, giving us a burst of courage and power to, say, jump into a freezing lake to pull out a drowning child.

But this response is often triggered when no one is drowning, the closest raging beast is in the zoo, and the only battle is in the boardroom. It's not a terrific background for living peaceably on a small planet crowded with other people who also anger easily. It doesn't seem productive to throw a spear at your boss or run away from your spouse, so, instead, you hold your anger inside.

The anger doesn't go away. The tension builds until it is out of control. Maybe you have an anxiety attack. You can tell someone off, but you know you will be sorry you did. You can hold it in, hide it, and feel ugly for even having such feelings. With no outlet for this chronic state of preparedness, you feel you are caught in a bind, may have to blow your top, or go into a blind rage. If you want to keep your job or your spouse, you won't give in to the impulse; the result can be an energy block, depression, or a serious physical illness. But it doesn't have to be this way. People can learn skills for expressing anger effectively.

Very young children are straightforward with their anger. They will just walk up and punch another child if they feel they have been treated unjustly by that child. As the child grows, she or he learns this is not productive behavior, and so finds other ways to communicate needs without becoming angry or learns to handle anger (appropriately or not) from the reactions of adults. The child may learn that anger is an excuse to kick a hole in a wall or hurt someone. Or the child may learn that anger itself is bad, embarrassing, something that nice people do not have, and would certainly never show. Not being able to handle anger appropriately can be very destructive.

Expressing other emotions, (guilt, for example is socially acceptable in the twentieth century but many still believe that expressing anger is not. Yet anger is often the only appropriate response to a bad situation. When people believe that it is not okay to express anger, they submerge it inside themselves. When this happens, issues that caused the angry feelings in the first place cannot be resolved because the lines of communication, for both pleasure and anger messages, are dead. All that is left is emptiness or indifference, which often breeds more anger. When people mask anger behind "nice" words, the listener gets a mixed message — anger expressed/anger denied — and feels an uneasiness; *i.e.*, "Do I believe the message you are sending, or the message I am receiving?"

What is communicated to children is: "Anger is bad." Or: "Nice people don't raise their voices." Or: "Showing negative feelings is low-class." Or: "Respectable people always maintain control." Children learn that open and direct expression of angry feelings toward another is a source of anxiety and embarrassment, so they learn to keep these emotions to themselves. Many people feel guilty for even having angry feelings and become masters at double talk, either denying the anger entirely or admitting only to a degree of it. Anger has many guises:

"I'm not angry, but I'm so tired of your behavior."

"I'm not angry. I'm just disappointed in you."

"I'm not really angry, but the way you are behaving is pretty disgusting."

But you *are* angry, so why say that you are not? Instead of saying it, you get your revenge in subtle ways by piling guilt on the other person. Or the hidden anger may become masked behind self-imposed martyrdom:

"How can you do this to me?"

"You should be grateful. I did it for you."

Sometimes the denial conspiracy is forced on to the child: "Don't tell anyone that Daddy and I have been fighting."

"I feel down today" is acceptable to say among polite adults who would never admit to being angry. It may indicate a passing mood, the fatique from carrying anger around, or a deep depression. The more extreme "I wish I were dead" is a cry for help.

So what has happened to you, the smart and prepared baby who was born with a healthy sense of anger, in the process of learning to conform to life in what we like to call civilized society? Did you learn to hold "need messages" inside, not to show the feelings that would help to get what is needed?

You may have learned the lesson of anger denial so well that you no longer even have the capacity to feel anger. You even may have learned to hide the feeling from yourself. This denial of angry feelings is like hearing a telephone ring again and again and cutting the cord instead of answering. The messages don't get through, even those that would give you pleasure. This is the price of efficient denial. Denial as a response to life creates difficulties in living comfortably with another person. Denial creates distance, and distance kills relationships.

Sarcastic and hostile comments are an example of "bound" energy of the passive-aggressive person. The energy it takes to behave in a passive-aggressive way could better be used to express honest feelings.[105]

Another destructive way to react to anger is to hide it behind a smile. We all know a Mr. Nice Guy who lets everyone else have their way. But no one can know him very well. He is distanced from us by a façade of dishonest feelings, the result of passive anger. Passive anger is different from aggressive anger, not in degree of angriness, but in the noise level. Both are equally angry.[106] Learning to express feelings honestly and to ask for one's needs to be met are the ways out of this syndrome.

Anger is a neutral energy. If stored, it can become toxic, both physically and emotionally. It can produce allergies and anxiety attacks. Out of control, it can destroy people. Used positively, anger can give strength, release tension, and generate warmth and good feelings.

The Anger Quiz

Think back to your childhood. What were the ways people around you responded to your anger? Were you expected always to "be nice"? Were you told "You shouldn't feel that way, it isn't ladylike/gentlemanly"? Were you punished for expressing anger? Were you told that you were "just selfish" and sent to your room? Worse? Did you receive any of the following "messages"? "No one will love me if I'm angry." "I don't feel it." "I shouldn't feel it." "I'm bad for feeling it." These are destructive messages. Check your present anger reactions with the following quiz:

1. When an unsettling event happens, do you feel anger right away?

2. Does it surface into your awareness only much later, after the fact?
3. Do you express your anger?
4. Do you hold in your anger?
5. Do you express your anger appropriately?
6. Do people get hurt from your anger?
7. Do you avoid blaming others?
8. Do you hold grudges?
9. Do you take the responsibility for the expression of your anger?
10. Do you expect others to "mind-read" your feelings?
11. Do you have a person with whom you can safely share your angry feelings?
12. Do you sulk or brood?
13. Can you turn your anger into constructive, well-used energy?
14. Do you smile when you are angry inside?

First draw a triangle around the even numbers of the answers you marked "yes". (Odd-numbered responses indicate more healthful and constructive approaches to anger.) Look at your even-numbered answers for areas in which you feel comfortable making a change. Write the changes you choose to make in this space: _____

_____

_____

_____

_____

_____

Making Choices About Anger

We do not have to be victims of uncontrolled anger and emotion. We can let go of the habit of thinking we have to become angry in order to institute change. One of the most effective techniques for taking charge of an explosive situation is to stay calm when everyone else is not.

Perhaps someone does something that bothers you. You become aware of your angry feelings and you need to make a choice. Is this a situation about which you really need to do something? Honesty is the way to be assertive with anger. Assertive anger says, "I have these needs. My needs are important. Is there a way my needs can be met without hurting you?" Stating our needs this way, with a question mark at the end, can clear the air. It gives the other person choices and opens the way for negotiation and the possibility of resolution.

In another situation you may decide that acting upon your anger will not serve your purposes. In some circumstances it may even be counterproductive. Combating sexism in the workplace may be one of those instances.

Mariette, an executive with a clothing chain, looks at it this way: "I think the most important thing on any job is never to take people's statements about you too seriously because you can drive yourself crazy, especially as a female in business, if you let everything bother you. Men will frequently say things that they don't even mean and things of which they themselves are unaware: sometimes sexual innuendos; sometimes something about your competency; sometimes a sexist remark. If I sat around and collected them all, I'd get nothing else done!"

Mariette is conscious of her anger energy. She knows what she is feeling and knows that she has choices about her response. She feels she can make a stronger statement with action than words. Dealing with sexism each time it happens, she says, would be energy-draining and counterproductive to her own goal which is to be recognized as a topnotch manager. For Mariette, then, achievement is "the best revenge."

Getting Free from Resentments

> It's a poor sort of memory that only works backwards.
>
> — Lewis Carroll

Putting anger into a creative project can be productive. Anger held too long, though, turns to resentment. Gretchen is a painter who can hold a grudge like Ebeneezer Scrooge held on to his halfpence. She remembers, collects, and preserves not only injustices but also slights and oversights from years before. Her art reflects her anger, so people don't buy it for their homes. This gives Gretchen something else to be angry about — "not being appreciated." Since her work is oversized and outrageous, the critics debate about it and the press loves it. An opening of one of Gretchen's exhibits is always a media event.

If Gretchen wished, she could dispel her anger productively through her art, but this is not what she chooses to do. Instead, subscribing to the "artists must suffer" school of thought, she wallows in her angry feelings, truly believing that without these hurts, her art would be nothing.

Strong emotion is valuable. It can be especially useful to an artist. Gretchen's problem is her resentment, her inability to forgive. She probably hasn't forgiven anyone for twenty years. Her anger is an energy that is stuck, unmoving, not connected to the world outside herself. Her life is very unhappy. Without forgiveness, the grudge hurts like a chronic ache in the bones. How do you forgive? You let go, you understand, you overlook, you love. As you pardon others, you yourself are pardoned. Forgiveness is the key to freedom from long-standing angers. By tying oneself to unhappy incidents long ago, the unforgiving person stays trapped in the past.

It's true, some people do things that are really hard to overlook. But you are not serving yourself by hanging on to a worn-out negative attitude. Martin Luther King, Jr, said, "Forgiveness does not mean ignoring what has been done or putting a false label on an evil act. It means, rather, that the evil act no longer remains a barrier to the relationship. Forgiveness is a catalyst creating the atmosphere necessary for a fresh start. It is the lifting of a burden or the canceling of the debt."[107]

Active forgiving can be a real opportunity for growth. Test these attitudes out on any old resentments you may have hanging around:

— What has this incident told me about myself?

— Why was this person (or situation) so adept at pushing my panic buttons?

— Could it be that this person (or situation) who is causing me all this agony and sleeplessness may have an important lesson for me?

Like us, our planet continues to suffer from our lack of the ability to forgive. Bitter resentments have been passed from generation to generation as though they were in the genes. Collectively the resentments have grown in many parts of the world into wars of long standing. Nations remain divided because of resentments that began so long ago that no one remembers the first incident in the struggle. On a planetary level, the need to forgive and start relationships anew is crucial — perhaps a massive emergency course in forgiveness will be our only chance as a species for survival.

Go ahead. Forgive somebody. What's stopping you? A mean little voice inside that says, "Why should I forgive those so-and-so's?" You have at least one good reason: because you the grudger is hurting more than the object of your resentment, the grudgee. Is the person you are resenting losing sleep as much as you are? Having aches and pains? Losing concentration? Why make yourself suffer more?

One of the people I talked to in preparation for this book spoke of taking the responsiblity for his resentment: "I may blame someone else who is standing in the way of my accomplishments, but what can I do? — Swear a lot at that person? Forgiveness is part of the healing process and I have learned that I am my own greatest obstacle. When I have let someone stand in my way, diverting my thoughts or attention, I realize that it's really not them, but it's me, getting in the way. When I give the anger a little time and distance — all necessary parts of the healing process — I can start to recreate that person's image and the image of our relationship more objectively. Looking at the positive aspects, when I get out from being ruled totally by my emotions, I see that it is never all positive or all negative — all me or all them. It's perception and attitude. The feelings will pass and I can help them pass."

Old anger is the waste material of the emotions. It's unhealthy to keep it around, clogging your energy source. Get rid of it, preferably in some constructive way, like the energy transformers in the following chapter.

Transforming Anger Energy

One person with a belief is equal to a force of ninety-nine who have only interests.

— John Stuart Mill

As a motivating energy, anger can be a very positive emotion. It has been the driving force behind great works of philanthropy, politics, and art. When put to its best use, anger can give strength and point direction. Many political movements sprang from collective feelings of anger (the Boston Tea Party, for example, which set off the American Revolutionary War.) Anger can be a great call to action, the impetus with which to transform energy into positive goals.

Val Prescott knows all about this.[108] "In 1967, when our doctor told us that our six-month-old son was blind, he said, 'I think children like that are better off in an institution.'

"When we drove home from Rochester that first day, Dick and I were so enraged at the doctor's suggestion that we did not even feel sorry for ourselves or our son. I'm sure that what a lot of people saw as our strength was our anger. Many people, when they learn that they have handicapped children, go through a period of grieving. We never did that. We had the attitude of 'We'll show him.'"

The Prescotts did not institutionalize their son as the doctor suggested. When I interviewed Val, her son John, who had become a gifted pianist, was playing a Chopin piece in the next room. A handsome and active young man, John was completing high school and was receiving offers from prestigious colleges nationwide.

John's accomplishments were not without effort on Val's part. Finding the best education for John had not been easy. Obstacles appeared and repeatedly Val rose up and fought. Val had to cut through bureaucracy after bureaucracy to obtain mobility training for John. She saw to it that he had Braille lessons even though it was necessary for him to travel by taxi between two schools. When one of the schools had a cutback in funds, eliminating the program that made it possible for him to attend, another school had to be found. At one point, it seemed there was no way the public school (that had some of the specialized services) and private school (that could handle John's other needs) could cooperate. Undaunted, Val looked at what her son needed and made it available. Val appealed to many sources, including the state board of education. She finally located a school for him that was ideal. John excelled there, eventually become a Carleton College National Merit Scholar.

When John's high school graduation day approached, Val realized it was John's leaving for college and his independence that she had been working toward for years. Not one to wallow in the "empty nest syndrome," Val took stock of her resources. She was well educated, had high energy, had experience with fund-raising and high-level leadership in volunteer organizations. "I know how to use the power structure as it exists," she said. She also knew how much help it had been that her husband, Dick, was a lawyer. "What happens," she asked, "to children with similar needs but fewer resources? What about blind children in other countries, where there are no talking computers, no books in Braille or on tape? Blind children whose fathers are not lawyers? What about the people in India who were blinded by the chemical accident?" Her energy, initially fired by her anger, was propelled now by recognition of a desperate global need.

With her interest in international affairs and the skills she learned as the parent of a blind child, she and her husband decided to start a foundation to help blind children in Third World countries. "I have learned that I have to look beyond my assumptions," she says. There are many countries with no services at all for the blind, Val explains, even to teach them to cut their own food, to learn basic coping skills.[108]

Talking to Val, one gets the impression that John Prescott's achievements are just the beginning — the training ground, so to speak, for this energetic and talented woman. She has found what she calls the right path for herself — the one that uses her skills and enflames her passions — in order to reach out from her family's needs to the needs of the world.

Expressing Anger

What do you do with anger that doesn't seem to lead naturally to creative action, that cannot be negotiated away or painlessly let go? Do you explode? Grind your teeth? Eat a whole bag of chocolate cookies?

There are other ways to release anger:

- Kick a can or a ball around a track.
- Talk to a trusted friend or a therapist.
- Go to the basement and scream — really scream!
- Meditate.
- Smash bottles at the recycling center.
- Ride a bicycle until exhausted.
- Yell at television commercials.
- Go for a ride in the car and roar and scream.

- Play tennis or other sports.
- Wash walls feverishly.
- Write a person's name on a golf ball and whack it around the course.[109]

Taking your anger out on an object can be more useful than holding on to the attitude "so-and-so has wronged me and deserves my anger." You may be perfectly correct about what the person deserves, but dwelling upon it isn't productive. No matter how angry you are, so-and-so really gets off scot-free, and you are left to seethe. Carrying the anger punishes you more than the other person. So discharge it by pounding on a pillow with a tennis racket or hitting a body bag with a whiffle bat. Some people play a piano or drums wildly, chop wood, or prune bushes to dispel anger energy. Take anger out on *things*, not people.

Be conscious about your anger decisions. Once you have your anger energy in a healthy place, you don't have to move a mountain in order to discharge it constructively. Here are more suggestions for dealing with anger:[110]

Find the Need Whenever you are angry, try to get to the underlying need: What do I want that I am not getting? Maybe what you need is something simple, like a hug, a listening ear, or someone's presence while you are going through something tough. Many times, if you can search yourself on a deep level and identify what you need and express it, someone will be able to fill it for you.

Identify an Angry Feeling While it's Warm By recognizing an anger response as soon as it occurs, you have greater ability to short-circuit the anger and turn it off before it gets too strong. If you express it when you feel it, it will not have a chance to build up inside.

Aim Well   Direct your anger toward the actual person who "pushed your buttons," rather than displacing it on to others, including yourself.

Don't Personalize   Sometimes we become angry because we think someone is deliberately doing something to us when, upon dispassionate evaluation, we can see that what he or she is doing may be merely thoughtless, not directed at us at all. Take a moment out immediately after you feel angry to sense the person's intention. Say to yourself: Am I *really* the target here? If I am, is getting angry worth it? Is there a better way to handle this person?

Show, Don't Vent   Some rules for negotiating through anger (formerly called "arguing"): 1). By stating what you feel (in sentences beginning with "I feel . . ."), you can transform a potentially anger-causing situation into one that can be successfully negotiated; 2). Be angry with the person's behavior, not the person; this way you can continue to love, honor, and respect the person while disapproving of the behavior; 3). Keep your statements in the here-and-now, rather than bringing up "history" — unhappy events or perceived injuries from the past that only stir up angry feelings; 4). Stay focused upon the outcome you want from the situation; 5). Avoid using sentences that start with "You . . ." when you are angry; 6). Accept the outcome. Even if you don't effect change, take pride in having been true to yourself and genuine with the other person.[111]

Write a Letter   When you are upset with someone, write a letter to that person, stating exactly how you feel, and then throw the letter away. You will feel better and you will not have made the situation worse.

Turn it Around   Ask yourself: What positive thing can I do with this situation? Poets, artists, and political cartoonists can readily use their anger as well as their positive feelings in their art. Novelists often get their "revenge" by creating characters out of someone whose behavior is bothering them. Many people have been motivated by anger to create great things.

Affirmations From Erik Esselstyn, Ed.D, and Micki Esselstyn, M.S.W.

- I am worthy of nurturing.
- I can get angry and still be okay.
- I love life.

Thought Replacements From Barbara Krebs, Ph.D

- Anger is worthy of me because it's part of me.
- Anger is a good honest emotion that can help me get more out of life.
- Anger is a signal to do something.
- I can live in the moment.
- Anger energizes me.

Affirmations for Resentments

- I never look back. My life moves forward.
- I choose to be happy.
- I send you, _____, my best wishes and warmest regards.
- I forgive you, _____, and bless you for helping me grow.

Step 7.   Handling Stress Productively

Stress is not the enemy. Stress can be productive, even necessary. Because relaxation is the flip side of the stress/release cycle, you could not even move a muscle without a little good stress.

What causes stress for one person may not cause stress for another. Riding a roller coaster is stress-as-excitement for some, but for others the experience is just painful. Mountain climbing, hang-gliding, moving from one home to another, speaking in public, getting married and bearing children are events that are stressful to some and exquisitely pleasurable to others. Some people are more stressed by boredom than danger. For others, change itself is a cause of stress. In most cases, it's not the stress-producing activities themselves that hurt us, but our response to them.

Stress occurs when we feel one way and act another. Imbalance, disharmony, and disconnection between body and mind are the result of being out of touch with our body's signals.

Stress Signals Quiz

Stress signals are one important way that your body has of talking to you. The more you have not listened, the louder your body will talk. When the signals change to mild symptoms, you begin to notice. If you do not act upon the stress message that the body is sending by reducing your stress level, the mild symptoms turn into illness. Then you are forced to listen.

Following is a list of the more common signals and mild symptoms, our bodies' initial and secondary reactions to stressful events. Check those that sound familiar:

_____ Your muscles ache.

_____ Your stomach hurts.

_____ Your head aches.

_____ You tap your feet.

_____ You grind your teeth.

_____ Your heart pounds.

_____ You reach for a cigarette.

_____ You reach for a drink.

_____ You feel hungry when you aren't.

_____ You get indigestion.

_____ Your hands get cold.

_____ Your neck gets tight.

_____ Your breath gets short.

_____ You catch a cold.

_____ You suddenly become accident-prone.

_____ You feel yourself breaking out in a rash.

_____ You make mistakes.

_____ You can't concentrate.

_____ You feel tired.

_____ You feel bored.

_____ You feel anxious.

_____ You feel confused.

_____ You feel frustrated.

_____ You snap at someone.

_____ You laugh nervously.

_____ You cry.

_____ You get depressed.

_____ You doubt your abilities.

_____ You feel like a martyr.

_____ You say something cynical.

_____ You don't care.

_____ You are too tired to get up in the morning.

_____ You forget something important.

_____ You lash out.

_____ You clam up.

_____ You go off by yourself.

_____ You feel lonely.

_____ You feel misunderstood.

_____ You feel unappreciated.

_____ You feel distrustful.

_____ You feel useless.

_____ You feel hurt.

Look at each item you have checked. Rate each one numerically, not by intensity of stress but by which stress reaction you perceive first, second, third, etc. By being aware of the first stress symptoms, you can respond to your body's call for some relaxation before your body needs to bring out the kettle drums and trombones in order to get your attention.

How does a stress signal show itself as a symptom?

- Fatigue. The body gets worn down.
- Work suffers.
- Ulcers result from excessive unrelieved stress.
- Anxiety, depression, and high blood pressure are some of the ways the body expresses itself when it is chronically stressed.
- Vulnerability to illness and reduced immunity to infection. Stress and how we handle it can alter our immune systems. Although the research on the cancer-and-stress connection is not conclusive, in multiple studies there appear to be links between stress, depression, and the immune activity of anti-cancer cells.[112] Studies have strongly supported the link between psychological factors and both the onset and development of infectious diseases.[113] The stress of college examinations had measurable impact on the immune systems of students in a Ohio State University study. Results included the body's reduced ability to produce interferon, which fights infection and disease.[114]
- The demonstrated link between stress and heart attacks has been accepted for a long time. New research has again confirmed this relationship.[115]

Knowing we can influence our own health to this degree gives us strong reasons to take control of our stress/relaxation response. Our thoughts, our inner imagery, and how we decide to react to an emotion can be considered a "chemical" in the way it affects us — the same as the foods we eat, drugs we take.

Instead of allowing our stress reactions to change our body balance in a negative way, we can intervene. We can change things by changing our thoughts, our emotions, our relaxation methods, the exteriors of ourselves, and the food/drug/environment level.

Taking Charge of Your Stress

Stress is detrimental when it is driving us, when it is outside our control, when it builds without a means of release. When we are in the driver's seat, staying balanced and in control of the stress and the relaxation, our energy is free to flow for — not against — us. Stress management is the art of taking control of our stressors and altering our responses.

The stress alarm sounds, and we may be aware of a thought, a physical sensation, a feeling of being off center or pulled in too many directions. In a normal stress situation, there's a period when the body recovers and returns to the normal state of relaxed alertness. If the ups and downs of alarm and recovery come too rapidly, the stress becomes chronic. The body never gets a chance to say "Whew!" and relax.

Maybe you don't let the "Whew!" happen. The following are chronic stress-producing situations:

- You try to achieve the unachievable or please the impossible-to-please boss.

- You try to make yourself fit into a role or love relationship that isn't right for you.
- You have too many tasks confronting you and no way to say, "Hold on. I have enough to do already."
- You struggle just to stay on top of things and never allow yourself (or are allowed) the feeling of accomplishment.
- You accept a promotion to a position you know you can't handle.
- You try to cope with the stress of work or family by retreating into alcohol or drugs.

If you see yourself in any of the preceding or similar situations, if you can recognize that you are setting yourself up for chronic stress, reassess. Is it time to level with your boss or mate and make some changes?

Employers are becoming more aware of the toll stress takes on employees and the advantages to the company of energetic and healthy workers. Some large companies have documented that stress results in physical problems and loss of work time. To compensate for this they have instituted physical and mental "wellness" programs, which help employees quit smoking, cope with stress, and make other life-style changes.[116] Union officials are starting to call wellness and stress management programs in the workplace a basic human right.

No matter how enlightened your own company or union and how extensive its concern, ultimately each of us is responsible for our own stress control. We are the ones who have the most to lose or gain, and we are the ones who must adapt ourselves to the changing world. We have choices about the stressors we will allow into our lives and how we will respond to them.

Numerous studies have shown that those who have a strong social support system are better able to make important positive life changes. Connecting to others and learning positive habits of interdependency are ways out of the stressor rut. A well-developed personality can take as well as give, need as well as be needed.[117]

Doing hatha yoga, learning relaxation or meditation, and developing healthier attitudes toward time and punctuality are useful stress reducers that are explored in detail in other parts of this book.

Workaholics

"It's hard to say what drives me. It's something inside of me — this unidentifiable object that keeps bugging me. It is what drives me toward my goals. It's a demon."

Donald is a flamboyant entrepreneur in the communications field and self-described workaholic. In spite of the tremendous drive he describes, Donald seems happy. While workaholics seem to be in an enviable position, as a group they are most at risk for burn-out. But Donald seems to have beaten the odds — so far.

"My drive is toward long-term objectives — multimillion-dollar business acquisitions — so there is no satisfaction right around the corner. I feel frustrated and thwarted because I want to accomplish more than is really possible. I would like to be less driven. Sometimes I wish I were happy having a job that demanded less of this, as it would lead to a more simplified life-style. But I love the challenge. If I had a less demanding job, I would be less driven, sure, but I would also be less interested.

"There have been times when I have had emotionally caused energy blocks. I'm talking about total block — paralysis, in an emotional, physical, and mental way. Because of emotional factors, largely. Once I had such emotional distress that I virtually could do nothing. Total depression. A frozen energy level. Zero capability.

"I have used various techniques to get out of this situation. In some cases I just take to my bed, not fight it. Sometimes I get over it by socializing with a friend. I get energy from my friends. Other times I exercise vigorously. Basketball, volleyball, racketball, hard vigorous exercise. The more vigorous, the more it takes my mind off what is on my back. Afterward, I can focus my energy on a creative solution, focus on the thought process rather than on the tenseness."

So far Donald has been able to pull back and recover. He has recently remarried and loosened up on his schedule. He and his wife have a new baby, who has charmed his way into Donald's life. Because the baby is helping Donald realize what is important to him, he is slowing down, spending less time spinning his wheels in what he calls his "brown-outs."

Many people who use the term *workaholic* to describe themselves are happy and productive people, but some social scientists believe that the obsessive drive to achieve is a sickness in itself, damaging the family and the organization as well as the individual.

Unhappy workaholics ignore the fact that they do not have unlimited time and energy. The usual workaholic response to stress is to work harder, which creates more stress. Donald has so far avoided this syndrome. For those who are caught up in their obsessive pursuit of achievement and success, there is no time for movies, music, nature, conversation, personal growth, affection, love or anything that isn't oriented specifically toward their goal. Some find that sex is more trouble than it is worth. Fantasizing, like emotion itself, is a threatening feeling because it carries with it a certain loss of control.

Unhappy workaholic executives fear losing control more than anything. The paradox is that, in the quest for more power and control, they lose the power to control their own time. In this sense they become like lower-level management people who experience high stress because they have little control over the ebb and flow of their work lives.

Happy workaholics are highly motivated because of a sense of commitment, not from fears or "shoulds." Happy workaholics are energized by hard productive work, and really love excellence. The difference between work and pleasure become blurred as more social life takes place with business contacts and more business takes place outside working hours. Business vacations become the norm. Happy workaholics are having fun on the job (although spouses may be suffering) and sometimes enjoy work more than play.

There are three strong antidotes to stress — a strong family support system; an active inner life; and job autonomy. These are Donald's strengths. The most important reason he doesn't burn out may be he has job autonomy. He sets his own goals, his own hours, and works at his own pace — a furious one, but it's his choice.

Many studies have shown that those who believe they have control over their lives can easily make healthful life changes. Taking control of your life is an inside job, not something that can be granted or imposed from the outside. Inner exercise, like affirmation or meditation, is the way to do it.

The Job Autonomy Solution

Numerous studies have found that the single most important factor determining job satisfaction is work autonomy, the degree with which employees feel they can make their own decisions and influence what happens to them on the job. A recent study indicated work autonomy to be as important as high incomes to the employees' job satisfaction.[118]

Giving employees more say in their work by dispersing decision-making power from the top down seems antithetical to the standard pyramid-structured corporations, but it has been found to improve productivity greatly. Flextime, worker-owned companies, quality circles, and work teams replacing the assembly lines are all ways to reduce job-related stress and motivate and energize employees.

Job Autonomy Quiz

Answer yes or no to the following:

• Is work flow determined by you?
• If work flow is out of your control now, can you take

steps to control any part of it?

- Do you determine your own hours?
- Do you determine when you take breaks?
- Do you decide when you go to lunch?
- Are you in charge of how fast or slowly you work?
- Are you in charge of what work is done first?
- Can you make changes in your physical work space?
- Is there a possibility that you can control more of the preceding factors in the near future?
- Can you specifically name one or two areas in which more autonomy can be yours now?

Study your answers carefully. Sometimes having more job autonomy is simply a case of taking more responsibilities for work as the opportunities arise. In other work situations, each change must be carefully and skillfully negotiated. Analyze your situation before taking action.

If you feel that you have some control over your work, your work environment, or your home life and if you have the confidence that you can rise to any challenge, you may be the kind of person who thrives on stress.

Skills for Coping with Stress

The regular practice of hatha yoga is my number one recommendation for stress. The following suggestions may also be useful.

Board of Advisors One way to make a difficult or stressful decision is to go into a meditative state and create a wise old character from whom you can ask advice. Donald, profiled in the section on Workaholics, visualizes not one person but a whole board of advisors. "Sometimes when I have embarked upon a particularly difficult project, or need some advice, I have conjured up certain advisors, wise men of my acquaintance, now dead. They are people for whom I had great regard and respect when they were living. One happened to be my father. I visualize them vividly and ask them questions."

Donald has not lost his mind and he is not having a séance. He has discovered what is becoming a highly respectable and effective form of inner dialogue. "When I got the answers and reflected back on it [the situation], I realized that if I had been able to ask myself the same questions carefully and in a relaxed manner — loose, not tight — I could have come to the same conclusions and that these answers may be a reflection of my own advice to myself, if I could do it that way."

Keep a Stress Log By becoming aware of your stress and keeping a conscious and methodical record of stressful situations, you may be able to avoid some and better handle others. Record not only the event but your feelings (including physical sensations) about these events, any statements that you say or want to say to yourself to dissipate any irrational thinking, and what other new action or new feeling of which you are now capable. Dr. George Krebs, in his workshops on stress management, suggests that you listen to your body systematically for one week, and every hour, if possible, take a reading. Ask yourself: Where do I feel stress? Where do I feel relaxed? What just happened? Within a week you will see a pattern that will give useful insights into handling stressful situations.

Once you learn the pattern of your stressors, use your calendar to schedule in moments to do nothing, time for art, music, fun, nature, loved ones — whatever relaxes you. Arrange more breaks, more vacations, time to savor your life.

Clarify Goals   Being clear about what you really want moves a lot of static out of your way. An example: When grocery shopping, you can reduce your stress level by knowing what is more important to you, time or money. If time is more important, you will be willing to pay more and whisk through the store in a hurry without reading the fine print. If money is more important, you will take the time to clip coupons and search out the bargains without resenting the time it takes. Once the basic decision is made, you are free of the tension of trying to be fast *and* thrifty. Identify other stressful conflicts (expedience *vs.* popularity; spending time with your child *vs.* time with your briefcase, etc.) Clarifying your basic goals will help you be decisive.

Sponge Up Relaxation   The simple act of lying on the floor on your back, palms up, feet 18 inches or more apart, letting the floor hold your weight, is rejuvenating. This is called the Sponge Posture in hatha yoga. Add some slow breathing for serious relaxation.

Cultivate Silence   Find moments when you hear only your own breath. Hear it, observe it, marvel at it.

Reduce Stress with Empathy   A helpful attitude to take toward the slow person driving in front of you or the indecisive person in line ahead of you at the store: They're doing the best they can.

Don't Sabotage Yourself   Ask yourself whether your stress response is helping or hurting the situation. Example: A young woman crashed her new sports car into a light pole in order to avoid hitting another car that pulled out suddenly at a blind corner. In the seconds after the accident all the bystanders expressed clear support for the young woman in the sports car — until she talked. In her stressed condition, she directed vulgar obscenities at the other driver, probably before she noticed that the other driver was a very old woman. Shocked by her outburst, the witnesses immediately and spontaneously switched their versions of the stories.

The young woman suddenly was perceived to be at fault, to be driving recklessly, traveling too fast, not watching the road. They held this impression and testified to it in court. The young woman didn't realize it was her reaction to stress, not her driving, upon which she was judged. (She lost.)

Play a Game and Plan to Lose Make up your mind in advance to lose. Then sit back and observe the pleasure of losing.

Quick Fadeout Close your eyes. Let the "screen" go black. Breathe in and out slowly. Sense your body. Ask: What am I feeling. What do I need? What can I do about it? Repeat one of your affirmations, like: "I can relax and let go." Fade back in. Continue your day.

Take a Walk Walking, like any exercise, can release a lot of tension. One executive who works for a multinational corporation walks to other employees' offices whenever possible rather than using the phone. These little walking breaks, he says, refresh him.

Rehearse Stressful Situations Take time to discover what, if anything, about your job causes fear — sales presentations, board meetings, writing memos. Mentally rehearse these situations, visualizing yourself handling each with confidence and assurance and bringing each encounter to a successsful close.

Unwind/Put Your Feet Up   One of the best ways to relax, especially if you stand a lot on the job, is to rest with your feet higher than your head. The most obvious way is to put your feet on your desk, although this is probably frowned upon in most offices. After the work day you can lie on the floor with your buttocks next to a wall and rest your feet above you on the wall. The change in circulation in your legs is both relaxing and energizing.

Visualization for Stress   The moment you realize you are stressed, stop what you are doing, if only for a moment. Breathe out a long breath and remind yourself that you are in charge of your response. As you do this, be aware of what your inner dialogue is saying. Does your stressed inner voice sound like this? *I can't do it. This is too hard. I'll never make it. I look bad. I can't handle this.*

Don't just take it from that negative voice inside. Argue. Talk back. Give back your rational best. Your strong self can argue like this: I can do it. I've done it before. I'm capable. No problem. I enjoy a challenge.

Wait until things calm down. Now change gears and take a mini-vacation. As you breathe out, visualize your favorite place, the place where you can best relax: your favorite fishing spot, the ocean, under a favorite tree of your childhood. Concentrate upon your visualization. Make the place as vivid as possible. Feel yourself relax. Enjoy the feeling. You know that you can have this feeling as often as you wish. As you practice this technique more, you will be able to land in this "vacation spot" sooner and with less effort. Eventually, you will be just a breath and a blink away.

Step. 8   Reconciling Time and Guilt

Supermom + Super Career = Super Guilt

Our society still believes nobody can raise a child like mother can. This may be true, but it's a puzzling stance for a nation in which nearly 50% of women with children under one year are in the labor force.[119] Although most employed mothers do not go out to work by choice, we have another contrary mandate: You are nobody without a career identity. Being just a mother is not enough for bright competitive women. But missing out on motherhood, many women believe, is missing out completely. So women are trying to be everything to everybody — the model wife, the nurturing mother, and the fast-track employee. Here are some of their voices:

Executive, Thirty-two, Married, Two Children: "There must be something wrong with me that I'm always so tired. Right now I'm too tired to cook dinner. I'm even too tired to go get some carry-out Chinese food. The kids need gym shoes, but if I go out tonight to buy them, I won't be able to get the report finished for tomorrow's meeting. My husband? He's still at the office."

Systems Analyst, Twenty-nine, Married, Two Children: "Time. I don't have enough for my child. I don't have enough for my husband. He gets what's left of me at the end of the day, and that's not much. Sex? That's a pleasant memory."

Real-Estate Lawyer, Thirty-two, Unmarried, One Child: "It's the emergencies, the unforeseen events, that are the hardest. I had to take my two-year-old to a five-hour closing because the sitter didn't show. It was a distraction, but the work got done. I decided not to be embarrassed about it. All the men at the meeting had children, too. What would they have done?"

Secretary, Thirty-nine, Divorced, Two Children: "I try to be both mommy and daddy to the kids and I can't. The kids blame me for the breakup. Some nights I come home and cry. Sometimes I think I'd like to get into the car and just keep driving into the sunset."

Teacher, Tutor, Cosmetic Salesperson, Forty-three, Married, Five Children: "I still have guilt about not being the best housekeeper, about not being the best cook, and not being the best decorator. I have the guilt of not excelling at those things because something inside still tells me that these are the things I really should be doing. That voice inside also tells me I should be enjoying them.

"I am the most tired and angry while I am cleaning the house. I have negative thoughts and remember things my husband did or didn't do five years ago. Yet I feel too guilty to be able to hire somebody to come in and help me even though I am earning enough money. I will never let myself think that I can afford it."

Art Dealer, Thirty-three, Married, One Child: "I'm really spread thin. This is not to say that I don't love my baby, it's just that I have a lot of guilt. I worry that my husband thinks that maybe I'm not a good mother, that I don't want the baby. It's not true, but I do get sick of talking to a baby all day. Yet I don't want to have somebody else raise him so that I can go out and pursue my career. I suppose I will do it in a few years, but I'm not ready just to walk out the door right now. The idea is not easy — that maybe all I am is a *mother*. None of my friends have babies. I have no one to talk to about this who will understand. People think it's blasphemous or something.

"Yesterday for the first time I went to a play group. I was like the wallflower at the ball. The other mothers were comparing prices of formula and diapers, and I was having an anxiety attack! All I could think of was; 'Get me out of here!' Of course, I stayed for the baby's sake.

"My business is doing fairly well, but I can't sleep thinking about how much better it would be going without a baby. I feel like I'm losing touch with what is new. My inventory of art is pathetic because I can't just pick up and fly to another part of the country for a few days. Things that were very easy for me, like making business phone calls, are much more difficult. I start the day earlier and work late, after he's in bed. I don't waste a minute. When he takes a nap, I dash to see how much I can do before he wakes up.

"I sound like I'm miserable and I'm not. I'm complaining, sure, but I worked hard for this career. The art world moves fast, and if I don't keep up, I'm out. Ultimately, I think that if I'm a mother who has a career, I will be more interesting for my child. I don't think it's healthy to throw your whole life into your kids. They grow up and then you have nothing."

This sounds like a no-win situation, doesn't it? Most of these women are exhausting themselves performing their multiple roles as responsibly as possible, yet they feel guilty about not doing enough. Some express feelings of guilt about slighting their careers, other about neglecting their families. Yet what I hear from mothers who are at home full-time is another kind of guilt — a fear that they are not growing, that their career is disappearing. This dissatisfaction is often expressed in the self-diminishing statement, "I'm only a mother."

This is the conflict of the decade and it will only be alleviated with more cooperation between the government and industry. It's happening — but slowly. Only a small percentage of employers offer child-care services (about 2,000 out of 6,000,000,000), but these are the giants, the pacesetters — I.B.M., A.T.&T., Proctor and Gamble, Campbell's Soup — and represent a national trend toward making child care part of a company's optional benefits package.[120]

There may be substantial improvements in the future. Policy makers are beginning to look favorably at such changes as substantial leaves for childbirth and infant care and income replacement for the duration and continuation of employee benefits.[121] Representative Patricia Schroeder said, "The superwoman has collapsed — collapsed of exhaustion. The work force has changed. It's time the workplace changed."[122] There's no denying that women need more flexibility in the workplace in order to be effective both at work and home. For those women on the fast track, it's not easy to resist the pressure to achieve early in their careers. Employed mothers can help themselves a bit by separating the time problem from the guilt problem. These are two different issues. People have roles to play *and* jobs to do. Jobs take time. This is a fact of life, so there's no use heaping guilt about it upon yourself as well.

Perhaps we need a different definition of *success*. The kind of career responsibilities that are possible at one stage of life may not be possible (or desirable) at another. The attention you can (or choose to) give to your career before you have a family and while raising small children may be quite different. In the future women may recognize and plan in advance for a three-stage career: pre-children; while raising children; and post-children. Many women use the second stage fruitfully to gain more education or new job training by working at part-time positions while the children are small. This, of course, is not possible for single parents, or when couples lock themselves into life-styles and large mortgages that require two incomes at this stage of life. The transition into the different career stages will be easier if given some planning and preparation. Start now. On a large piece of paper, draw a projected "life line" for your future, including what you expect from yourself, your family, and your career in each year until you retire. Be sure to include the year and the children's ages and needed income for each year of your projection.

Another solution is for fathers to take equal responsibility in the family. Can the father take turns staying home when the kids are sick?

The fathers with whom I talked want to be with their children more than they feel their jobs allow. The big difference that I hear from men is that while they regret not spending more time with their children, they accept the job as a necessary fact of life (as it is for most women who hold outside jobs) and thus aren't as ready to fall victim to the guilt. An executive and father of two, who tries to attend all his children's school athletic events, every play, and every piano recital, says, "Sure, I want to spend more time with my kids. I suppose I feel a little regret about not being able to, but I don't feel quilty about the very fact of working. Sure, the kids can lay a guilt trip on you. You don't have to accept it."

Goodbye, Supermom

It seems that for many women, the word *mother* translates into *housewife*. One who distinguished the difference early is Linda Hoeschler, forty, wife, mother, and group vice-president of her company. I was about to believe that perhaps motherhood no longer exists without guilt when I renewed my acquaintance with Linda.

"I guess I feel that no matter how supportive and helpful my husband is, I always feel the emotional burden is mine to make the household run smoothly because I like a clean, organized house. I want the children to be all they can be. The way that I cope with it is to hire a replacement for myself at home. I don't want to come home from work and do grocery shopping, or cook dinner (even though I like to cook), or fold clothes or iron or do the laundry or clean the house or weed the garden. So I hire people to do that. That allows me to not do the part of the supermom job that I don't like to do."

Linda says she feels no guilt at all about hiring people to replace her at home. She accepts the responsibility for certain jobs, for the primary care of the children, and for the organization of the house without an emotional investment. "I have always tended to delegate. Maybe it was because I was the oldest child and was treated like a son, so to speak. From the time I was a very young child, both my parents told me that I should be able always to take care of myself, that I should figure out a career, know how to handle money, know how to get a job, that I should never be dependent upon anybody else for anything. Because of that I acquired a certain belief in the need to be self-sufficient. Being able to delegate is part of that belief.

"I think that I saw my parents delegate things, and trust other people. I used to be kidded as a child. People use to say, 'Linda could delegate going to the bathroom.'

Even then I would go around to people who didn't appear to be busy and suggest things they could do. Now my leadership lies in the fact that I am able to effectively utilize people's talents and skills, and that I am able to get people to work together to do things for me and like doing it.

"Sometimes I overdelegate. I try to walk a fine line of doing what I need to do to learn all the details of the business, but when I have all super people under me, I would just as soon give it all away."

Delegating means giving up some control, and that is true in the home as well as at work. Linda is undeniably in an enviable position; not many career mothers can afford the kind of help she has. Yet it could be argued that her career success may be due in part to her attitude. With adequate help and no burden of guilt draining her energy, she can give 100% to her job during the day.

Linda's confidence stems from a firm understanding of her own independence in relation to her role in her family and growing up with an independent mother as a role model. As women gain more experience with power outside the home, they can trade off some of the burdensome power within the family, and become strong role models for the next generation.

As women give up control in the home, men take on more. A study in 1981 indicated "a wide-ranging adoption of emerging values by married men as they accept non-traditional family roles.[123] The study, conducted by Benton & Bowles, Inc., demonstrated that men now asssume a wide variety of tasks once considered to be women's work: 32% of the husbands surveyed reported shopping for food; 47% cook; 29% do the laundry; 28% clean the bathroom;

and 80% in households with children under twelve help with the child care.

The study also found that 62% of the men interviewed said they believe "the family is stronger" if husband and wife share responsibilities, including providing income for the family. But 70% also believed a contradictory statement: "Unless it's an economic necessity, a family is better off if the woman of the house does not work." Apparently, it is not only women who have conflicting feelings on this subject.

Things to Feel Guilty About
(For Parents)

Choose which answer best describes you for each category:

HOUSEKEEPING

_____1. I feel guilty that I'm not a better housekeeper.

_____2. I like my house to be tidy and well kept. I feel guilty because the children don't feel comfortable playing without worrying about messing up or breaking something.

_____3. I'm emotionally neutral on this one.

THE JOB

_____1. I worry that I don't spend enough time on the job. Or: I got a promotion I don't deserve.

_____2. I spend too much time on the job. Or: I got a promotion; therefore, I feel obligated to spend more time on the job.

_____3. I've got this one under control.

THE BRIEFCASE

_____1. I bring home work to do at night and on wee-
    kends; therefore, I must be slighting my family.

_____2. I don't bring work home; therefore, I must be
    slighting my job.

_____3. I've resolved this issue.

CHILDREN'S HEALTH

_____1. I feel like a nagging parent, trying to get the
    kids to brush their teeth, or eat right, or not
    smoke, (if they're older).

_____2. I should be more involved in my children's
    health.

_____3. I've/we've resolved this one.

THE RESIDENT HELP

_____1. The children are taking more of the burden
    of the housework than is healthy.

_____2. The children don't help enough. They should
    learn responsibility.

_____3. We've come to a workable agreement on this
    issue.

MEALS

_____1. I spend too much time on meal preparation
    and not enough time with the children.

_____2. The children should learn about good food, but
    I don't have time to prepare it, so we eat a
    lot of junk. I know it and I feel terrible about
    it.

_____3. We eat simple, nutritious food. Everyone is well
    nourished and this is not an issue.

MY TIME

_____1. I feel guilty when I take time from the family
    for my own hobbies or exercise.

_____2. I resent that I never exercise or have time for hobbies.

_____3. I've balanced my life between time for myself and others.

CHILDREN'S CLOTHES

_____1. The children are becoming too materialistic and clothes-conscious. I should spend more time teaching them wholesome values.

_____2. The children aren't stylishly dressed, which reflects badly on my role as a parent.

_____3. I've found the balance.

OTHERS' ACCOMPLISHMENTS

_____1. My spouse didn't get an expected promotion. Maybe if I had been more supportive . . .

_____2. My children are doing poorly in school. Maybe if I were home more . . .

_____3. We are all responsible for ourselves.

Check your answers. The #1s and #2s are more active issues for you. The #3s that you marked indicate issues that are resolved, at least for now.

Energists have a cool, realistic pragmatism about what is and is not possible for themselves and what does or does not serve their goals. They don't berate themselves for failed dinners and unmade beds. Aware of the limitations of a have-it-all life style, they maintain control over what is possible and let go of the rest. They don't diminish themselves by emulating impossible role models. The bottom line in a given situation is: How much does this matter to me?

Look at each active issue you marked in the preceding quiz and ask youself the following:

- Is the answer I gave based upon real facts, or does it stem from habitual guilt?
- If these are the facts, can I do anything to change them?
- If I cannot change this reality, can I do anything to change how I feel about it?

Choose *one* that is an issue with you and upon which you are willing to take action. Write below one step you can take *today* to disentangle yourself emotionally from one of these issues. What we feel emotional about rules us. What rules us drains energy from us. So separate your emotions from your jobs, rules, and identities. A little healthy detachment can be energizing.

_____
_____
_____
_____
_____

Time Use

Time can be passed, wasted, spent well, lost, found, given away, speeded up, slowed down, stretched out, waited out, bought, or borrowed. But not matter how you use it, twenty-fours hours a day of it is all you are allowed. Heads of state, beach bums, beauty queens, and employed mothers don't get more of this elusive commodity than you do.

True energists are aware of the quality and use of their

time. Wanting to live fully each waking moment, they do not let time casually slip away from them. Effective use of time can be accomplished serenely as well as frenetically.

James Boen, Ph.D., Professor of Public Health, Specialty of Biometry (the mathematics and statistics of health research) at the University of Minnesota, is very aware of his use of time. When I asked to interview him, he and his wife, Dorothy, a manager of materials and distribution for a health-maintenance organization (H.M.O.) and a fine violinist, invited me to dinner.

Jim learned effective time management from necessity after an accident. When he was nineteen and a junior in college, Jim, a body-builder and gymnast, broke his neck at the sixth cervical level, while working out on the horizontal bar. The accident left him a quadriplegic, in a wheelchair, although through rehabilitation he has limited use of his hands and arms.

"I was a very proud young man. The energy source for my rehabilitation was a social anger — anger at the condescension I was receiving. In the early 1950s in the Midwest, the social role for a person with a disability as severe as mine was to be a perpetual convalescent, handicapped, a disabled person. I felt I was to forever play the patient role, which is to be constantly cheerful and grateful, to cooperate with all treatments, take everyone's advice, receive their patronizing and condescending behavior. That was very repulsive to me. In terms of compensating for the loss of my body, I discovered that I could still learn, and that while I was not a brilliant mathematician, I was adequate. So I went into mathematics."

Unwilling to play the role of the patronized victim, Jim struggled to learn the skills he needed to live independently. He learned to feed and care for himself. He drives a specially adapted car and commutes to the university from Hopkins, Minnesota, where he and Dorothy live with their two children, now college-aged. Jim has done volunteer work with disabled children and adults, including Vietnam veterans. He has helped initiate programs in sex and drug therapy. He has traveled alone nationwide to do consulting or lecturing. One of his hobbies is hunting. He has successfully bagged bear, elk, deer, antelope, caribou, and jackrabbits.

Jim's limited physical energy and strength require that he pace his energy and use his time extremely well in order to maintain his successful career and active life. He does this with the same intention and decision-making that energized his rehabilitation. (A person dependent upon a wheelchair must spend more time doing things the rest of us take for granted: getting in and out of cars, waiting for elevators, planning routes that avoid curbs, stairs, and places inaccessible to wheelchairs.)

Jim and Dorothy are efficient planners. While Dorothy can afford to leave more to chance, Jim schedules carefully, consciously, and decisively. He knows in advance the time and energy an activity will take and budgets accordingly.

Jim says that the place where most people waste time and energy is with "social shoulds." "I very selfishly avoid wasted time or actions, especially wasted social interaction. When I'm on a committee that isn't going anywhere, I simply resign, and tell them why. I don't go to a social function I would not enjoy if it is at all avoidable. I don't invite people over simply for social obligations. I just don't bother with the normal social amenities that people don't need — like small talk — that are just time-filling."

Jim says that most people simply are not aware that they have a wide range of choices in social interaction. If there is something else a person would rather do, it is possible to decline and simply not participate. Jim believes that people too easily fall victim to things they don't want to do. They use "shoulds" as excuses to avoid taking responsibility, or to feel self-righteous about the activities they think they are compelled to do, or to justify their chronic fatigue. They don't exercise their choices; they can't say "No."

Jim gives an example: When he and Dorothy have guests and he doesn't want to stay up and socialize any longer, he says, "Okay, my energy is run out. I'm going to bed now. Good night."

A lot of people wouldn't be able to do that. It takes a certain amount of courage to go against social convention. Jim responded with a twinkle in his eye, "It would be a problem for me, too, if I worried about whether people like me. That is not one of my problems."

Although Jim has freed himself from social obligations, he still must pace himself carefully. "I like to exercise, so if I have extra energy at the end of the day, I'll use it to exercise. I would rather do this than engage in a lot of small talk. . . ."

Perhaps his dry sense of humor balances his nonconformity. When he and Dorothy give a dinner party, as they did the evening I was there, it's a lively event. Since

Jim eschews small talk and extending obligatory invitiations, the company and the conversation are extraordinarily interesting.

Time Use

You own your time and energy. You are not obligated to give it away against your will. Are any of the following areas ones in which you could gain energy by relieving yourself of social "shoulds"? (Some people are energized by casual social contact. This quiz is for those who are not.)

- Do you attend social functions when you'd rather be elsewhere?
- Do you continue relationships that no longer offer you growth?
- Do you do *anything* for "old times' sake" (unless you are sentimental and enjoy this)?
- Do you serve on committees whose functions you doubt, or for which you have little interest or commitment?
- Do you do anything because its hard to say "no" to people?
- Do you entertain people you don't enjoy?
- Do you make small talk of more than four sentences?
- Do you continue love relationships after you know they aren't going anywhere?

Consider your answers carefully. Ask yourself if your handling of these situations represents your honest choices or "shoulds" that you could be happier without. Resolve now to lose those time-gobbling "shoulds." When you give your time and energy to others, give it willingly and joyfully — because it's your choice.

The Case of Near-Fatal Listmaking

"I just don't have any pep. However, when I'm doing something that I feel is important, I'm the original driven woman. I'm a snail today — I can't get things done. Why am I always tired? Was I born tired? The days I have energy, I will try to get through all those lists I have made. I'll run here and there and check things off on my list and keep going and going. Then I'll collapse and vegetate until the cycle turns around again."

Alexa and her husband live in a contemporary house of her own design. Their children are grown. She has a high-pressure job in sales, has exhibited her art, and is a sought-after member of the community for spearheading drives and creating social change. Concerned about the fatigue, Alexa had a physical. The doctor tested for anemia, an underactive thyroid gland, heart problems, and diabetes. Everything checked out okay. She investigated the question of allergies. She was already taking vitamins.

I asked Alexa how she accomplished so much in spite of the fatigue. She said, "I'd be lost without my lists. I'm always making lists. I have my main one next to my placemat on the table, so that it's handy to refer to. I feel great satisfaction from crossing this off, crossing that off. I have lists all over the house. Lists for house-cleaning jobs, groceries, things to make for the children and grandchildren. I have lists for errands like the dry cleaner, and things to buy. A list for letters owed to people. I put my hobbies on the list as well. Things I want to do someday if I have the time, something new to take up next. I have a long-term list: 'Things I Want to Take Up.'"

You wouldn't expect people to die of making lists, but Alexa came close. Alexa had lists down to a fine art. For efficiency, she was without equal. Her trouble was that she expected herself to accomplish everything on her lists. There were no optional items. For her, the list became not a suggestion or a reminder but a command.

Like the executive workaholics who respond to stress by working harder, Alexa kept trying harder. When she felt she was not accomplishing enough, she made a longer and more efficient list that would necessitate her working harder to accomplish. When she became fatigued, she tried to become more efficient by doing two things at once. She scheduled activities that would normally be thought of as relaxation or recreation into her schedule as though they were duties, something to add to her list of "shoulds."

One night after our interview, Alexa was rushed to the hospital. She underwent emergency abdominal surgery for peritonitis. Had she lived farther from the hospital, or if the surgeon had not been immediately available, Alexa would have died. The dramatic events surrounding her sudden, near-fatal illness shocked her into taking stock of her life-style and her priorities. When she realized how much she expected of herself, it became apparent even to Alexa why she was tired. There were more tasks on the lists than she could have put into two or three people's schedules.

She has a different job now, and a new attitude. "I allow myself to not do two things at once. I still make lists, but I ask myself first, 'Do I really want to do this?' Sometimes I don't, so I leave it off. I also don't worry if everything on the list is not accomplished.

"There's one more change I've made. I don't know if it's just superstition, but the nature of my illness seemed connected to my long lists. So after that bout with peritonitis, I decided to take better care of myself, especially my gastric/digestive tract. I no longer keep my lists next to my dinner plate."

Time Savers

Time and energy spent keeping our living quarters orderly can drag us down, but so can living in a disorganized environment. Here are some housekeeping ideas from energists who would rather be doing other things:

- Use an egg timer when you clean house, allowing three minutes per room. Or decide that you will do the whole thing in a certain amount of time, with some reward after that.
- Put on a peppy record and dance through the house, cleaning as you go.
- Hire yourself to clean at the same rate the cleaning service would charge and use the "mad" money for things you normally wouldn't buy.
- Motivate yourself by inviting someone to your home and decide that you will have it clean before this person arrives.

- Display a large chart listing chores to be done and allow the children to choose. The choice factor encourages more cooperation than an assigned job.
- When accumulated tasks seem endless and overwhelming, tape a large piece of butcher's paper to the wall of your kitchen and break all the big tasks down into manageable parts, followed by the estimated time each would take. For example, "Clean the House," a big job, can be sliced into forty or more parts, like "Sort left-side drawer, three minutes," or, "Wash kitchen window, one minute." This way you can cross off an item or two while waiting for an egg to boil or a child to appear for lunch. These minutes seem like freebies, and they help diminish the magnitude of the larger job. Remember to leave something on the list for tomorrow.[124]

One full-time housekeeper discovered that she rather liked cleaning but really became bored, even despondent, about cleaning her own house. So she started a cleaning service, managing a crew to help her clean other people's houses. Some of the money she makes is used for paying someone else to clean her house! There's always a solution. It just takes some imagination to find it.

How to Distinguish Depression from Fatigue

To have ups and downs in your energy level is normal. It's a way to grieve, to recover from problems, to wait before taking action. But it's not easy to distinguish between normal ups and downs, the fatigue that comes from plain tiredness, and the fatigue that is part of serious depression.

In *mild fatigue* there may be a lowered attention span, a lot of vague complaints about life, poor muscle tone. If the underlying reason is other than disease, eating better, exercising and getting out among people more (like doing volunteer work) may help, along with other suggestions in this book.

Chronic fatigue may be a response to everyday stresses: time pressure demands; worry; family problems; monotonous work; unresolved emotional conflicts, just to name a few. These signs all too easily mask true depression. Because the body and the mind are intertwined, symptoms like fatigue are not so easy even for the physician to diagnose. This situation is further confused by the tendency of people to use the term *depression* when they mean they are not as energetic as usual, or they are in a bad mood.

Chronic fatigue can be brought on by long-standing insomnia, by lack of exercise, by undereating and the current craze to be bone-slim. But overeating and carrying around a mountain of extra fat can cause fatigue as well. Some chronically fatigued people often work longer hours than required.

True depression involves the total person; the changes are physiological as well as psychological and include every system in the body: nervous, endocrine, digestive, cellular.[125] The sexual urge is often affected and the emotions may be in a state of paralysis. The chronic depressive often feels self-critical, hopeless, uninterested, unmotivated. Signs often include cynicism, indecisiveness, getting upset over trivial matters, hostility, becoming excessively obsessed with guilt, or being unable to express anger, even if there is a hurricane of emotions whirling inside.

The chronic depressive needs professional help. A medical doctor is best qualified to make the determination. If you are really feeling down — to the point where life doesn't seem worth living anymore — pick up the phone and get a professional on your side. You're worth it.

Energy Pacing

One energetic entrepreneur told me, "I have to be really alert and able to concentrate when doing important creative work. It is almost like taking a magnifying glass and focusing the rays of the sun into a very bright hot focal point. I find that in order to do that, I have to conserve my energy and not waste it on a lot of details. I really try to store it up for major creative thought, strategy, and plans."

The following are suggestions for your energy pacing:

Rest   Knowing when to rest is as important as knowing when to push. More breaks are better than fewer. Researchers believe that two or three in the morning and afternoon are optimal.[126] If you usually take a fifteen-minute break each morning, see how three five-minute breaks work. However, if you are doing physical work, more food breaks are necessary to replenish calorie expenditure.

Effective resting is more than simply changing pace or drinking coffee. Meditating or exercising for a few minutes (especially if you can do it out of doors) is the best way to perk yourself up for the rest of the day.

Being Your Own Permission Giver   You don't need someone else's permission to take care of yourself. Don't wait for the stress crisis to relax. Don't wait for total exhaustion before taking a nap. A fifteen-minute catnap or meditation break while you are still functional can pick you up readily. If you wait for the crash, it may take you all day to recover.

Finding a Devoted Companion   Being able to relax with "unconditional love" can make you feel more energetic. Where can you find someone who will love you as you are, be devotedly loyal, give unlimited affection, and never criticize or argue? At your local humane society! Stroking and talking to your dog or cat can actually lower your blood pressure![127]

Protect Yourself from Intrusions   Do what it takes: a secretary with the instincts of a bulldog, a phone-answering machine, etc.

Say "No"   When a proposal is made that will take your time and energy, make it a habit to *stop* before you agree. If you need time to think, say so. If you are on the phone, use this old trick. *Say* "Hold on while I check my calendar." *Stop*. Put the receiver down. Close your eyes. Ask yourself, Do I really want to do this? What's in it for me? (If you have an extreme case of "yes-itis," ask yourself, If I had three hours left to live, would I choose to spend it this way?)

Give yourself time for the answer to appear. You may get a "Yes, that would be fun." You may decide you would learn something worthwhile, meet some interesting people, get to know an acquaintance better, or derive some other advantage. Whichever way you answer, *let it be your choice.*

Remember: *You don't have to give a reason.* If the person asks, switch to the offensive: "I'm surprised that you'd ask." or: "Why do you want to know?" If the person doesn't get the message, you can always resort to a simple "no." Now congratulate yourself on the hours you have saved to devote to something *you* find important.

Finding Time

Inevitably, some of the best-laid plans go awry and well-organized calendars require adjustments. Even the most efficient planners sometimes find themselves waiting: a plane is late; the supermarket line is long; traffic has ground to a halt. Using this time productively eliminates some of the stress of feeling that the time is wasted. I call these instances *found time.*

Be Prepared   Carry a small book that you have been wanting to read, or some articles cut from the morning's paper or your journal in which to record your dreams. Open your pocket calendar and plan the next week, month, or year.

Socialize   If you are with someone, get to know your companion.

Go Inside   If the place is quiet enough, meditate. Enjoy being alone. Observe the quality of the silence.

Play Movie Director   Observe those around you and ask yourself: What if . . . What if your favorite TV personality walked into this situation at this time? What if police chased robbers through this scene? How would people react? The possibilities are endless. You can enjoy a movie-in-your-mind by making up a scenario using available "characters" and moving them mentally into a story of your own making. Mind games or day dreaming can be very relaxing.

Let a Child Entertain You Ask a child to tell you a story or a dream. It will not only be interesting to you, but may open the youngster to the riches of the inner self. Only one story-telling session with an interested adult could be a significant event in a child's life. If the child is reluctant, be more specific. Ask if he or she knows any stories about dogs. Or ghosts.

Deep Breathing Only a few moments of diaphragmatic breathing can relax and rejuvenate you.

Listen to Audiotapes Get an audiotape player and leave in your car tapes of lectures, your favorite music, or tapes of your children talking. This makes long traffic tie-ups almost enjoyable. Commercial tapes are available on almost every subject from novels to medical journals. However, *never listen to meditation tapes in a car on the road*. "Going out" while driving could be fatal and I am always surprised to learn that some people, in an effort to be time-conscious, do this. People who love life don't need to be *that* efficient.

Examine Your Feelings Alicia, who does freelance word processing in her home, often found herself working into the night to meet deadlines, declaring she "didn't have enough time." At my suggestion, she tried Word-Spinning on the words she used to complete this sentence: "The largest and most unnecessary time gobbler in my life is —. She finished the sentence with the words "getting

ready to work," so these were the words she used for
WordSpinning. She found the reasons for her inefficiency.

To gain awareness of what role your emotions play
in your time management, complete one of these sentences:

- The largest time gobbler in my life is _____
- I would use my time better if _____
- When I'm very honest with myself, I know that
  my obstacle to better time use really is _____
- The way I could save time is _____

Now WordSpin your answer. What did you learn? What
surprised you?

Affirmations for Time Management

- I enjoy planning and mastering my schedule.
- I have confidence in my ability to make choices.
- I can handle everything that matters.
- I enjoy being efficient.

Step 9. Enhancing Self-esteem

Energists are central in their own lives. They balance the demands on them with their own needs and desires. They feel in control of the world around them. They trust the voice of the inner self.

In our culture we are not taught to trust ourselves. We look instead to authorities of various kinds to tell us how to live, work, play — even eat. Lacking this strong center of trust, we are vulnerable to perfectionism, shame, guilt, envy, excessive competitiveness, fear of failure, and general feelings of being undeserving — not a very conducive way to invite energy into our lives.

Remember "What you love grows"? In the beginning of the book we discussed the "love phenomenon": What we love and give our attention to grows in direct relationship to how much we love it. Whatever we have that needs growth or improvement needs first to be loved.

Before we look at how some energists solved self-esteem problems, ask yourself this: Are you loving yourself enough to develop self-esteem and give yourself an energy priority? People who love themselves are personally powerful. Self-esteem and confidence are like fuel in the energy machine. When we're out of self-esteem, we run out of energy as well.

Envy

"Comparing myself to other people bothered me a great deal in the past. I was expending an awful lot of energy wondering, worrying, asking myself: What am I doing wrong? How come I don't have . . .? And how come I don't know? I could have climbed Mt. Everest and I would not have been satisfied. I always wanted more."

Bright and dynamic, Kara had a successful career in the New York theatrical world. Yet, despite her considerable success, she never felt fulfilled. She was, in her words, "a high-energy person who wasn't harnessing the energy productively."

When Kara's energy ran down, she realized that she had been spinning her wheels trying to be and do everything that others were and did. She allowed what she observed about others to become the standard by which she measured her own life.

Envy can be debilitating. Since envy involves a comparison of possessions, achievements, or personal qualities, it is different from its sister emotion, jealousy, which usually refers to relationships that are threatened. Both "green-eyed monsters" fall easily upon those of shaky self-esteem, when the perceptions of others' achievements and abilities are personalized and distorted into feelings of personal failure. It isn't the other person's success that causes the trouble; rather, it's the unjust comparisons made by the envious person.

"What I envied about people was that they seemed successful. They had the outside circumstances I thought I wanted — the large houses, the vacations, the wonderful clothes, the large dinner parties, the Hamptons, Europe. Their lives looked happier, more successful, more full of accomplishment. I wanted to do and have the things that I thought gave satisfaction to these people. I had great goals. One was to go to New York and work in the entertainment industry, so I did that. I thought that was going to do it. I thought that relationships and three marriages were going to do it. I was still looking for the outside circumstances to give me inner peace."

Kara learned to turn her envy around over a period of time. As she recognized the envy as misdirected energy, her natural vitality returned, but with new and positive direction. With reflection she found that she would not really want someone else's life at all. Now, instead of saying to herself, I want what she has or I want to be her, she studies her subject like a scientist with a slide of microbes: What makes this person tick? What kind of attitude does she project that makes her so awfully attractive? Is her work or style of dress something that I could incorporate into my own life and enjoy? How would she handle this difficult situation?

When Kara identifies traits in others that she admires, she looks inward. What part of me is like (or unlike) that? What in myself could respond to more of Suzanne's elegance, or Margery's passion for sailing? Thinking it over, she decided that it was Suzanne's gracious self-confidence, rather than her clothes, that she coveted. Since Kara hated the water, she realized that it was Margery's passion, rather than her sailboat, that she enjoyed.

"I am no longer envious of anybody doing anything. Now I'm going with the flow and it's very peaceful. I don't know how to descibe the form of this new energy. It comes from a joy that's inside of me — a joy that I love life. I celebrate moment by moment just being here. I feel like a light inside of me glows from the joy."

Perfectionism

> I would not dream of belonging to a group that is willing to have me for a member.
>
> — Groucho Marx

Perfectionism is a peculiar kind of stress. For perfectionists with low self-esteem, the stress can be difficult. The "cannots" and self-doubts can grow into a huge and sometimes incapacitating energy block.

Often the perfectionist doesn't have the confidence to enjoy everyday living. The motivation for every activity is not the joy of doing it, but fear of failure. Many of the people I interviewed told of their struggles with perfectionism:

Cynthia, a talented actress and director: "I have been incapacitated, immobilized for years, because of thinking I'm not good enough. When I was younger, I would do many things without a lot of thinking in advance, and what I did would be wonderfully well received. But in the last few years, fear holds me back. For instance, it can take me all day to write a letter.

"I've been working on this with my therapist and I am now coming to the point where I can write a letter without thinking that it has to be the most brilliant, most literate letter. In situations that are not important, laboring over a letter to make it perfect just doesn't justify my time and energy. All I have to do is send the letter and give them that information. My new advice to myself is, 'Don't think. Act!'"

Nurse: "I've come to realize that my perfectionism was my way to avoid marriage. I kept my standards so high that no man was ever able to measure up. This kept my ego safe by allowing me to reject him before he rejected me."

Retired teacher: "Perfectionism can be crippling. I don't bake a cake because I'm afraid it won't turn out perfectly. I didn't make a phone call because I was afraid of the rejection. I love birds, but I didn't buy one that I loved because I was afraid that it would die."

Administrator: "My son William said recently that he could never do anything right to please me. I was stunned that my perfectionism has made him feel this way. I remember feeling that way with my parents. I had hoped that I wasn't doing that with him. But evidently I had."

Working mother: "I like my home neat and tidy, but I'm not a perfectionist in the sense that I would do a white-glove test on it anymore. But I like a certain amount of order around me. My husband will tell me, 'Relax, it's not important.' But I can't."

Manager: "One thing I have to watch when managing people is that I can't always expect everyone who works for me to get the same amount of work done in the same time and to the same standards that I apply to myself. I have had enough work experience in good corporate settings that I can make judgments really quickly. Other people take longer to do it. The older I get the better I have become at not expecting everyone to keep up with me. I have learned to say, 'This is what I would like to have done. When do you think you can complete it?' It makes me a more effective manager."

Math teacher: "I used to be a perfectionist. I used to think that I could be married, have a lovely home, hold down a job, and work on a master's degree. That madness ended after my first child was born. Now I have become less and less of a perfectionist, and I like myself more." She patted the side of the sofa affectionately. "Years ago a sofa that looked like this would not have lasted in my house one week. Now it has stayed here looking like this for months and I really don't care about it. What difference is it if the sofa is tattered? It's more important for me to do other things.

"Now my philosophy is: Calm down and enjoy life; it goes so fast. Sometimes I have been so intent upon getting things done that I don't sit back and take the time to enjoy the moment. I am moving now in the direction of achieving that balance between getting something done, having the energy to do it, and then sitting back and enjoying it. That has to be the best of all worlds, to have the balance."

The recovered perfectionists I interviewed spoke most often of repairing their self-esteem as the most valuable move they'd made away from the perfectionist trap. Like Cynthia, some had professional help. Several had a life crisis that led to change.

Sybil, a Texan who is now head of her company, had her turning point at a life-enhancing seminar. "In my first seven years of marriage, my negative energy was keeping me from a career even though I didn't know it. I was home taking care of the kids and I was trying to have the *perfect* children and the *perfect* household, always trying to keep my husband (who had always been the *perfect* son) *perfectly* happy.

"Worrying about what my in-laws thought prevented me from opening myself up to my own possibilities. I was always trying to please them (in spite of the fact that my husband didn't care at all about the stuff). They could never be pleased simply because I was not a relative. All my energy was going into hating them. What made the breakthrough for me was going through the Omega course, hearing its founder John Boyle. He said that energy can be directed positively or negatively.

"Until I went to Omega (that was twelve years ago),

I could remember everything I had ever done wrong in my whole life. In first grade I spoke out of turn in class and in third grade I cheated on a multiplication exam. I can still remember, but I no longer punish myself by saying, What an awful child I was! The affirmation "I never devalue myself through destructive self-criticism" was what changed me. Now I say it every single day.

"I realized that if I just put my energy into positive things I wanted to achieve, I would go so much further. I decided my goal was to get a job, and I affirmed for it. It was only a few months and I had my first job. Now I really don't care too much about what my in-laws think about me. I think they like me more, but I really don't waste energy on it."

When Sybil put her energy into a positive direction by working on herself instead of her relatives, her life changed. She learned that self-criticism has no positive purpose, that it's not the same as being realistic or making a logical assessment of weaknesses and strengths. It's fine to know what your limitations are. Then you don't have to let them limit you.

The Turkey Tradition

The trouble is we're taught to be terrified to make mistakes. That's especially true of Americans. Our flies have to be zipped, our hair always in place. We have to make sure we always use the right fork.
— Stephen Birmingham[128]

Perfectionists are often tangled up in rules, believing that there is only one perfect way to perform daily tasks and that there is someone out there — Mother, God, or the Keeper of Perfect Standards — who cares about how we perform life's little details. In fact, there are about as many ways to complete any task as there are people who would do that task. There are often good reasons to follow certain established routines. But sometimes we are just in a rut.

A new bride preparing to roast a turkey was struggling to cut off the tips of the wings. Her knife wasn't very sharp and at one point in the struggle both the turkey and the bride almost landed on the floor. A friend who was watching asked the young woman why she was cutting off the wing tips. The bride said, "Because my mother did."

Her friend's inquiry made her curious, though, so the next time the bride saw her mother, she asked her why she cut off the turkey wing tips. Her mother said, "Because my mother did." Fortunately, the bride's grandmother was still living. She made a special visit to her grandmother to ask why she cut off the tips. The grandmother said, "Because I have a narrow roasting pan."

The moral of the story: Question authority.

Procrastination

Procrastinators also suffer from low self-esteem. The procrastinator fears judgments, criticism, holds on to impossible standards, and sees any imperfection as failure. Procrastinators have a variety of styles. Rita's is what I call *brinksmanship*: "I have been a procrastinator all my life. I don't start a project until a few hours before the deadline.

Then I do everything in a furious hurry. I think that I like feeling the pressure. The pressure both makes me feel important, and relieved — relieved of having to do the project methodically and to the standards that people expect from me."

Rita doesn't believe that her best effort is good enough. In an irrational twist of thinking, a procrastinator like Rita waits until the last minute in order to have "permission" to complete the work. When time has run out she can finish, because she rationalizes that because of the time pressure, lower standards will be used to judge the quality of the work. Procrastination serves to prove to her that this work will not have to be a reflection of her true ability, but only how well she can perform under pressure. The result is the face-saving statement, "I could have done a much better job if I had only had more time."

Procrastinators avoid taking a stand, making a decision, completing a job. Others use procrastination to rebel against authority or to advertise their high standards.

Brad, who plays the role of the *connoisseur*, is one of the latter. He is a writer who doesn't write, a carpenter who doesn't build, yet he takes great pride in high standards. Brad believes his friends expect his writing would be superb and his furniture splendid. Brad is only fooling himself. Although he prides himself in his good taste, the reality of all his perfectionism continues to exist only in his mind.

His energy is totally bogged down in the details of a hundred or so unfinished "beautiful" projects. He has collected the finest cherrywood to build a table, which he has not built because he's "waiting for some old-world stain." Maybe he will take a quick trip to Austria for it sometime, but now his fine table appears to be a pile of boards among the other unfinished projects in the shambles that passes for the living room. His friends like him in spite of his fear of accomplishments, disorganized life, and chaotic apartment. They do not share his fantasy about his high standards.

Like other procrastinators, Brad is a master of the alibi. The deadline — the feared moment of judgment — is postponed this way, but the procrastinator is usually the only one that this illusion fools. Here are some other alibis:

The Exception claims, "I am a very punctual person who is never late, but this time circumstances out of my control caused my tardiness." In reality, The Exception always knows exactly what time it is and how close to cut the time because The Exception never wants to be the one kept waiting. The Exceptions are often not procrastinators at all, but manipulators of other people's schedules.

The Professor intellectualizes. Reasons for lateness go like this: "The prehistoric world had twenty-five hours in each day instead of twenty-four. I'm still running on 'prehistoric time.'" The Professor's excuses usually bear no relation to the real reasons for lateness and are designed to deflect attention from real or imagined inadequacies.

The Waiter waited for inspiration and it arrived late. "You don't want me to turn in something that isn't first-rate, do you?" It's hard to tell this exhausted, red-eyed alibi specialist, who lets you know that he stayed up all night to finish the project, that he just has.

I call Beverly's alibi style, *Duty Before Pleasure*. A gifted painter, Beverly has her basement full of huge colorful canvases — all unfinished. "I love to paint," she says. "Painting is my soul. Every morning I wake up and say, 'I'm going down to my studio right after breakfast and finish the still life, . . .' but I find something else to do first. I get caught up in cooking, marketing, ironing — things I really hate but think I have to do first. Before I know it, the day is gone. I busy myself with so many other silly things that I never paint. It is almost as if I punish myself this way."

Beverly hasn't made art a priority in her life. Instead, she has allowed keeping house by her perfectionist standards to become a dawn-to-dusk job.

Many people describe themselves inaccurately as perfectionist when they insist on quality work, or as procrastinators when they have overscheduled themselves. To qualify as real procrastination, the delay must be irrational and the condition must be chronic.

The number-one remedy for procrastination is to raise your self-esteem, to learn to trust yourself and your capacity for good work. Giving up unrealistic ideas of perfectionism is part of the change, in addition to replacing these ideas with achievable goals. Even the most determined procrastinator can make some progress when self-esteem is expanded.

A good first step is to learn to separate product (the job, the artwork, the project) from the self. The truly dedicated procrastinator may need professional help.

Loving the Holes in Your Socks

> When a man says that he is perfect already, there
> is only one of two places for him, and that is Heaven
> or the lunatic asylum.
>
> — Henry Ward Beecher, 1887
> Proverbs from Plymouth Pulpit

As a hatha yoga teacher, I often ask people to remove
their shoes. Once someone asked, "What if we have holes
in our socks?"

At some time, we all have "holes in our socks," some
little imperfection we'd just as soon not advertise about
ourselves. Our only mistake would be to believe that others
don't. All of us know in our heart of hearts that we ourselves are not a finished product. There is always room
for improvement, a little hole somewhere that could use
mending — or a tiny asymmetry that sets us apart. We're
never without something left to work on. (The root word
for *perfect* comes from the Latin and means *finished*.
Who wants to be finished?)

It's what I call a *perfect system*. As my practical Wisconsin grandmother used to say, "Isn't it funny that only
your favorite socks get the holes?"

The old sage, George Bernard Shaw, once said, "If
you have a skelton in your closet, you may as well make
it dance." So dance, sing, find something unique in yourself
to celebrate. There is, you know, something that makes
you unique among human beings. Letting go of ideal-
ization and perfectionism by fully accepting and loving
your glorious (and imperfect) humanity is the way to come
really alive.

Martin Buber, the existentialist theologian, suggests

that recognizing uniqueness in people is how one gets a glimpse of God. Following that line of reasoning, it would appear that hiding your uniqueness (flaws, weaknesses, fears) behind perfectionist conformity is not allowing others to glimpse the divine (perhaps also the human) in yourself. Perhaps we aren't judged so much by how well we have succeeded in life as whether we have succeeded at being our best self.

Reliving the Good Times

Choose a peak positive experience, such as when you were singled out for recognition for some good work. This can be something you were proud of doing yesterday or in third grade when you won a spelling bee. It is not important whether the deed was terribly important to anyone else, but how you felt at the time. It's these good feelings we want to recapture.

Do you have your incident in mind? First, relax and close your eyes. Use one of the relaxation methods discussed in the section on relaxation. You may want to read this into an audiotape recorder so you can hear the instructions as you go. Count slowly from zero to five. (You can say to yourself, When I reach five, I will be relaxed and ready for this visualization exercise.)

Slowly now:

1. See your incident vividly.
2. Who else is present?
3. See the environment in great detail.
4. See yourself as the honor is announced, the award being granted, the goal accomplished.

5. Feel what you felt then — the glow of accomplishment, of confidence, and self-esteem. Feel this in your body as well. Capture and enjoy this feeling.
6. Take a few moments here to reexperience this pleasure.
7. Let the feeling go, knowing that you can recapture it any time you choose.
8. If you wish, repeat one or more of the Affirmations for Perfectionism from the list below or the following, which is from seminar leader Martin Bronfman: "I love where I am. I love who I'm with. I love what I'm doing." [I add, "I love who I am."]
9. Slowly come back to your outside awareness by counting backward from five to zero. Tell yourself that when you open your eyes you will feel alert, energetic and ready to get on with your day. Begin to move, stretch, and open your eyes.

Doesn't this feel great?

Affirmations for Envy

- I love myself unconditionally.
- I enjoy being my own work of art.

Affirmations for Perfectionism

- I trust myself.
- I never devalue myself with destructive self-criticism.[129]
- I can think for myself.
- I can do the job perfectly but I don't have to.

Thought Replacements for Perfectionism

- I am not my work; my work is not me.
- My best is good enough.

Step 10.   Loving Your Body

There's a lot of "fat talk" going on. Have you witnessed any of the following exchanges?

When greeting one another, instead of inquiring about the other's health, some women now attempt to compliment others by noticing (rightly or wrongly) that others have lost weight since their last meeting.

Skinny person, greeting another: "Hi! How you doing?"
Other skinny person: "I'm fat. I put on half a pound this month."

Little fourth-grade girls overheard talking about their diets and their "ugly flabby behinds"? (If a 1986 study by the University of California at San Francisco is to be believed, about 80% of fourth-grade girls (in that city) said they were dieting.)[130]

Fat has become a national obsession, a multimillion-dollar industry, a great waste of energy, a health hazard, and a boring topic of conversation.

What's going on? Why does everyone want to be bone-thin? In one study, about one-third of the participants (more often women than men) were strongly dissatisfied with their bodies. Women more often than men were obsessed with their size. Often the women who feel badly about their bodies can be quite attractive, but don't believe they are.[131]

Other studies show that both men and women tend to be unrealistic about how others view their bodies. The difference is that men tend to think they are more attractive to others than they really are, while women view themselves as less attractive than others actually rate them.[132] This distorted self-image is especially apparent in regard to body weight and size. Women often feel fat and continue dieting even when they have become dangerously under-weight. The fashion industry has taken notice and resized clothes to provide for a "size zero" — for women who cannot bear to be a 2, 4, or 6. Isn't this the ultimate in the minimizing of the physical self?

Fortunately, a healthier, well-exercised look is supplanting the gaunt and bony look. But, rather than embracing this new energetic and athletic style, many of the chronic dieters I see are hooked on dieting, "fat talk," and guilt. (They feel guilty about every forkful they put in their mouths.) Their energy is diminished, not only by insufficient nourishment, but by battle fatigue — the war between themselves and their bodies that keeps them feeling anxious at meals, and depressed, deprived, and continually guilty in between.

Of course we want to look good. It's energizing to look good, so let's look the best we can. Becoming a walking skeleton, however, is not the same as looking good, feeling vibrant, bursting with life. Designers have encouraged this look for their own purposes. Yet many of us have become so intimidated by this that if a garment narrows where the body widens, we believe the body is wrong, not the designer!

If you look good naked but not in your clothes, the answer is not to reduce your size so that you can wear anything that the stores have the audacity to sell, but to learn to select clothing that brings out the best in your natural build. Wear clothes. Don't let them wear you!

If you have already decided you will not be bullied by unrealistic fashion images and that health and vitality are more important to you than looking like a famine victim, you're already ahead of the game. Hooray for you! Rejoice in your advanced consciousness.

Why Crash Dieting Is Useless

The whole idea of crash dieting is counterproductive to good health and good feelings. The word *diet* itself makes me feel deprived. When I feel deprived, the next thing I think of is the word *refrigerator*. The term *weight loss* isn't any better. It makes me think of Godiva chocolates.

Don't get me wrong. I'm not going to defend fat. Fat causes all kinds of problems, interferes with exercise, and makes us more prone to certain diseases. Carrying too much fat around is certainly a physical energy drain, but the national obsession with imagined excess weight is not exactly energizing either.

Who put all this emphasis on weight, anyway? Although *overweight* is what people commonly talk about, I prefer to say *oversized* because who really cares what you weigh, except for you, your scale, and your doctor? Size is what shows. Size is what determines whether you fit into your clothes. (If they are becoming tighter, you're becoming larger.)

Weighing yourself can give you a distorted picture. Your poundage alone cannot tell you if you are losing fat, water, or muscle. (Muscle weighs more than fat, so you *could* be building muscles, losing fat, looking slimmer, and gaining weight at the same time. This would be progress in the right direction, but your scale alone could give you the opposite message.)

It's muscle tone, not weight, that determines whether you like what you see in the mirror. The way to decide whether you are larger or smaller than your ideal is to take off your clothes in front of a full-length mirror and look. Is your flesh firm? Are you well proportioned? Muscular? Bony? Soft and begging for exercise? Are there bulges here and there? (You can estimate muscle tone by looking and feeling, but fat can fool you for a while into thinking it's muscle. Your doctor can measure this if it's important for you to know. If you are exercising regularly and rigorously, you know you're building muscle.)

The trouble with dieting is that it leads to more dieting. Crash dieting is a state of temporary deprivation, both physical and psychological, which eventually perpetuates the fear of food experienced by bulimics and anorectics.[133] Crash dieting keeps you preoccupied with the symptom level, which is not where the action is for permanent change.[134]

Crash dieting is the enemy of your metabolism. Two weeks of crash dieting can change your delicate metabolic balance and make subtle changes in your muscles that make you feel tired. You don't want your muscles to suffer — this is the part of you that burns calories. According to researchers, crash dieting encourages both long-term weight gain and high blood pressure — exactly what you don't need if you want to be vital and energetic.

Once you are finished with your diet, you may feel that you have earned the right to eat again. You may eat only a little, but your weight zips right up to where it was before, wiping out all your hard-earned gains. If you want to become a larger size, go on a strict crash diet. The end result of sharply reducing your natural caloric intake is that you will eventually gain more weight — not right away — but in a month or a year, or whenever your body starts to fight back.

Here's why: Proponents of the set-point theory believe that healthy people have an innate mechanism that guides the body back to regain the amount of fat it usually has.[135] When your metabolic system is healthy, it signals appetite control, energy level, and interest in vigorous activities. Ailing and rebelling, it can create feelings of lethargy, low energy, hunger pangs — whatever it needs to do to pull you back where you started.

One explanation for this is that while you were eating so little, your body learned to get along on very little. You body adjusted to fewer calories by reading the dieting pattern as a signal that there was a famine going on.

Searching back into its genetic coding, it retrieved the information that the way to survive a famine was to use the existing food very efficiently. What made sense years ago in times of real famine only causes havoc today with the body that is subjected to on-again, off-again crash dieting.

Another reason to avoid dieting is that it causes stress. Stress causes overeating in rats, and probably in humans, too. The brain's natural opiates, the endorphins, play a role in weight regulation in people and animals.[136] Under the double burden of excessive stress and unnatural eating habits, the body loses the effectiveness of its natural regulators. Nicotine and caffeine also interfere with the natural high we can enjoy when our endorphins are working with us. Many believe that the high incidence of smoking in teen-aged women is the result of stress caused by social factors and systematic food deprivation. The nicotine acts as an artificial compensation for a stressed metabolic system.

The answer to all figure improvements is not starvation but getting in touch with your body, owning it in a positive way, and nourishing your muscles with health-building food and exercise. Not harder exercise, but proper exercise, more often. Add walking for one-half hour each day, or riding a stationary bicycle for twenty minutes each day. (Add something you do not normally do in your regular exercise program.) Avoid fatty foods and eat a large percentage of your calories in fruits, vegetables, and whole grains. The results are not necessarily quick, but they are safe and assured. In addition, by following this plan you will have good muscle tone, which is more attractive than skin and bones, and a well-stimulated metabolic system as well.

A healthy metabolic system is the key to the whole thing, the genie in the lamp, the difference between a lusty, vital healthy self and a lifetime of deprivation, stress, and calorie counting. If your metabolism still works, guard this delicate mechanism, nurture it, and cherish it. Feed it right and bless it regularly. If your metabolism is ailing, nurse it back to health with good food, exercise, and professional help.

The "Why I Eat" Quiz

Sometimes we need to become aware of when and why we eat. Check the sentences that have meaning for you.

_____ I eat when I'm hungry.

_____ I eat when I need pampering.

_____ I eat when I need mothering.

_____ I eat when I'm frustrated.

_____ I eat when I'm bored.

_____ I eat when I'm angry.

_____ I eat to get back some nourishment when I have been nourishing others.

_____ I eat for revenge.

_____ I eat because I'm lonely.

_____ I eat because I really want sex.

_____ I eat to avoid having sex.

_____ I eat to punish other people.

———— I eat to avoid ever having to look well.

———— I eat to reward myself for good behavior.

———— I eat because the food is there.

Look carefully at your answers. Is eating the best solution? Use your answers to start a dialogue with your body. Next time you feel hungry, go to the source. Ask your body what it really wants. Then try to find a way that is honest and nondestructive to satisfy it.

The real reason to eat is because you are hungry — hungry for food. So, when the cue comes that signals you to eat, stop and ask yourself what you really need. Ask yourself, Am I hungry, or do I have an appetite? Choose between the two. If you have an appetite, it means you need something, but this something is not necessarily food. Knowing the distinction between appetite and biological hunger is the highest priority for a person with disturbed or compulsive eating habits. When you decide that food is not what you really want, avoiding food does not feel like deprivation.

There are other ways to deal with all of the afore-mentioned "appetites." Therapist Loretta Lewis, M.A., M.S., suggests the following:[137] If you need pampering, try a hot tub. If you want mothering, arrange to have a massage. If you eat to fill the time, try exercising the time away. Walking or riding a bicycle helps frustration. Racquetball is a good sport for discharging anger. Jumping on an indoor trampoline changes your mood, as does moving to music. Hatha yoga and t'ai chi are calming. The act of chewing itself is also soothing for ruffled emotions. Crunchy, chewy food like carrots, green or red peppers or celery sprinkled with spices can serve as aggression tools for calming yourself.

When you need emotional nourishing, phone a supportive person who you know will say good and pleasant things to you. (We can't expect everyone to love us, but let's seek out those who do when we're down.) If long-standing revenge is your reason for eating, consider that the best revenge is to live fully and energetically in the moment. An affirmation for this is "I'm taking care of myself and living fully."

Even when you are alone, treat yourself well. You're worth it. You can enjoy food on more than a taste bud level. Eyeball your food before you eat it. When you sit down to unwrap fast-food packages (or, worse, stand at a counter), you have only food as fuel, nothing else. Your whole system of sensation feels deprived. In contrast, you can feel satisfied on much less if you slow down and consciously enjoy the beautiful colors, tastes, textures, aromas, and pleasant surroundings. This sensate feast allows you to leave the meal feeling good, not deprived, and you will be sated with much less actual food. Learning to luxuriate in things other than food, such as beautiful table settings, is another way to satisfy a need without adding calories.

When sexual need is the reason to eat, it helps to recognize alternatives. Sexuality is a positive energizing force that doesn't necessarily have to be acted upon by making love or eating. Sexuality gives us the impetus to do other things like high-priority creative projects, such as athletics and dancing. There are non-caloric alternatives to overeating or inappropriate sexual behavior.

If you have life problems to straighten out, start now.

If you eat to get back at a parent, or if you don't eat to get back at a parent, straighten things out at the source and quit punishing yourself with symptoms. If you are chronically and obsessively hungry for anything other than nourishment, recognize this, and separate it in your mind from the whole issue of food and deal with that problem.

Do you eat because you are lonely? Or because you are alone? Don't confuse the two. *Alone* means you choose to be by yourself. If you are lonely — not alone by choice — you have other options, such as going to the movies, calling a friend or reaching out. Look for alternatives.

Next time you have appetite rather than hunger, choose an energizing activity instead of reaching for food. Others have worked their way out of this trap. You can, too.

Eating Disorders

The American Psychiatric Association classifies anorexia nervosa and bulimia as eating disorders. Anorexia nervosa is a serious illness of deliberate self-starvation with profound psychiatric and physical components. The symptoms of anorexia nervosa are: loss of 20% to 25% of body weight; lack of menstrual periods, hyperactivity, distorted body image; and food binges followed by fasting, vomiting, or using laxatives. Bulimia is a group of behaviors that becomes an obsession characterized by recurrent episodes of binge eating followed by self-induced vomiting or purging with laxatives and diuretics. Bulimia sufferers may be of normal weight, underweight or overweight.

One characteristic of both disorders is misguided

achievement orientation, so it is no wonder that it appears often on college campuses and even in high schools across the country. On the University of Wisconsin-Madison campus, the writer of a recent doctoral dissertation determined that 13% of the undergraduate dormitory women suffer from bulimia.[138] (However, men can also have this problem.)

The symptoms of bulimia are: inconspicuous binge eating; menstrual irregularities; swollen glands; frequent weight fluctuations due to alternating between binging and fasting; and the fear of the inability to stop eating voluntarily.[139] Most bulimia sufferers who have these symptoms experience a painful and irritated larynx and esophagus from vomiting. They may pass out because of severe vitamin deficiencies. Sometimes the esophagus ruptures, which can be fatal. Bulimia can also cause immediate death because the body's electrolyte balance is altered critically from vomiting.

Bulimia sufferers often know that what they are doing is not healthy and normal, and try to to hide it, but bulimics and anorectics may have a distorted notion of reality in regard to their own bodies.[140] Anorectics typically believe that they are fat, even when emaciated. They deny the symptoms, even while looking into the mirror. Many women caught up this struggle have lost the ability to see this syndrome for what it is. They actually believe that they are beholding beauty when what they are witnessing, in fact, is a deterioration into a possibly fatal condition. This battle for control spirals downward into a struggle of the self against the self. Once this cycle is firmly established, it becomes self-perpetuating.[141]

Bulimia and anorexia are difficult to diagnose, and

many sufferers display a combination of both illnesses. Eating disorders indicate a need to reconnect to the body and to respect the wisdom of the body's messages. This is not a do-it-yourself project. If eating disorders are interrupting your life, seek professional help immediately.

The "Love Your Body" Exercise

Changing habits is hard. If you love yourself, it's easier. When your body is with you, you have one less obstacle in your path toward energetic living.

Whatever you decide to do regarding your diet, start with loving your body. I hear you say, "I can't possibly do that. How can I love all this flab?" Okay, start with something about yourself that you like. You have nice eyes. You keep your nails beautifully manicured. You have a great smile that lights up the room. You have beautiful feet.

If you can love your body (or even part of it), you can enjoy eating wisely, exercising often, dressing well. Eventually, your body will respond to your loving attention and become more alive and vital, toned and more flexible.

The following exercise is designed to be done in the time you are taking a shower, while you are sudsing your body. You'd be doing that anyway, so you may as well add the inner exercise. As you lather your body, bring each body part to your attention with words that give positive messages. Say the words out loud if you can. Just follow whatever procedure you usually do while you shower, only bless each part as it is brought to your attention. If there are some parts you don't feel good about, say something neutral like, "This is my knee." Repeating "This is my ugly knee that I've hated since third grade" is not productive. Concentrate upon function, not appearance.

It's probably best to proceed in whatever order you usually wash yourself. As you continue sudsing, acknowledge each part of yourself in the same way. The following phrases are only examples, so make up your own words and don't get the book wet:

- I love my head. My head contains my magnificent brain.
- I love my face. It contains my senses of sight, taste, and smell. My face is the main way I communicate with others.
- I love my ears. I love hearing music, other people talking.
- I love my neck. It allows me to look from side to side. It supports my head.
- I love my hands. They allow me to _____. (insert the names of the activities you love most to do with your hands.)
- I love my arms. They allow me to reach beyond myself toward new accomplishment.
- I love my underarms and all the systems in my body that keep me cleansed.
- I love my chest. My chest protects my heart.
- (Women) I love my breasts. They are a source of pleasure. They nourish(ed) my babies.
- I love my abdomen. It contains my vital organs.

- I love my back. It's strong and it's flexible.
- I love my buttocks. They make sitting comfortable. They have cushioned me.
- I love my genitals. They are a source of great pleasure.
- I love my legs. They are strong legs and help me to be strong.
- I love my feet. They support me and carry me where I want to go. They are good, strong feet.
- I love my toes. My toes help me to be _____ (graceful, athletic, or some such appropriate adjective).
- End with an overall self-esteem builder:
  I love myself unconditionally.
  I am loving myself more every day.
  I bless my body.

(Are you questioning the use of the word *bless* in the context of this exercise? One of the meanings of the word *blessing* has no religious connotation. It means "to give approval to." A variation of this exercise, called "body scanning," can be done silently in a relaxed state instead of in the shower.)

Perhaps you aren't ready to love freely all of yourself. Women, especially, have a tendency to believe some parts are too big or too small or have imperfection. Many of us have scars or parts missing. These can be recognized positively as reminders of accidents we have survived or mementos of times that could have been worse.

Note which parts of yourself you have avoided in the exercise. Are these parts that also give you trouble in other ways? Parts left out of our conscious approval often are those most vulnerable to problems.

So what will happen to you if you start to love your body? If you feed it only the best food, if you exercise it regularly, if you pamper it as though it were a new lover, and if you bless it regularly as though it were the universe's personal gift to you — which, indeed, it is — what will happen?

The New You

People who have a greater perception of their control over their environment and themselves not only cope better, they have fewer health problems all around. Having choices helps people feel more in control, which by itself reduces stress and increases available energy. The following are areas in which you can take control of your body:

- Love yourself and enjoy your body.
- Rid yourself of food-related guilt and fear; be informed about which are better food choices, and gradually make more of these choices part of your everyday habits.
- Do regular sweat-producing exercise and be aware of your body's needs.
- Make deep breathing a habit. Conscious deep breathing connects body and soul, so to speak. Shallow breathing functions to set real feelings apart from us. Learning to fully and habitually take in good breaths helps you give and receive emotional feelings.

- Reduce your stress levels.
- Increase your feelings of being in control of other areas of your life.
- Develop new coping strategies (such as the ones in this book).
- Find a support group. Group therapy is effective for dealing with eating disorders and body-image problems.

* The suggestions in this Chapter are not intended as a substitute for professional intervention in cases of eating disorders.

The following are words to replace negative inner dialogue.

Thought Replacements

- It's okay to say no.
- I love my body as it is now.
- This is good nutritious food, full of life energy. I want this goodness to become part of myself.
- Who's in charge here, anyway?
- This food is worthy of me.
- I'm eating this because I love me.

Affirmations for Body Image

- I am free.
- I love myself unconditionally.
- I choose to have an attractive body.
- I love who I am.
- I can be whatever I want to be.
- I deserve to look good. I deserve to feel good.

Step 11.   Conquering Fears

It's easy to be brave at a distance.
—Aesop

Are you afraid of speaking in public? Flying? The dentist? Heights? Spiders? Elevators? Disease? Closed spaces? Storms? Certain animals? If you claim any of these, you have a lot of company. These are common fears, yet no two of us have quite the same list. Fears like these are energy gobblers.

Fear doesn't have to be an antagonist. Depending upon how we view it, fear can be a useful energy source and may even be one of our more helpful emotions. Fear protects us from everyday dangers. As children, fear of pain helped us learn not to fall from high places or to ride our tricycle faster than we could control it. Fear urges us to plan ahead in order to make our lives more predictable. It prompts us to keep our attention on the road when we are driving. Fear is what comes and taps us on the shoulder to say, "Hold on. Look before you leap. Is this what you really want? Do you need more information before you can take action confidently?"

The important thing is not whether a fear is reasonable, but whether it interferes with your life. When fear becomes excessive, worries become chronic and anxiety appears to rob you of energy. Let's look at each of these. *Worry* is an anxious style of dealing (or not dealing) with fears that nag at you. The source of *anxiety* is usually a general feeling of apprehension, rather than fear of a specific object or situation. Anxiety often manifests itself in physical distress. *Fear* usually is associated with a specific situation or object. *Terror* is an extreme, debilitating, and uncontrolled form of fear.

Do you remember the little gadget called the Chinese finger trap? The harder you try to release the finger, the more impossible it becomes. Only by letting go, by pushing counter to the direction in which your escape seems apparent, can you free your finger. Many of us fear finding ourselves in situations from which we cannot return but rarely are decisions so rigid that we cannot go back and choose again in a new set of circumstances.

As Pogo said, "We are confronted with insurmountable opportunities." Also, we are confronted with irresistable opportunities. Risk-taking appeals to the adventurer in us. We will continue to take calculated risks because we don't want to miss the possible successes waiting along the road ahead. Successes, even little ones, motivate us to pick ourselves up after events that are less than successful and try again.

Worrying Efficiently

> The trouble with Archie is he don't know how to worry without getting upset.
>
> — Edith Bunker

Everyone harbors a little caution about something, whether you call it fear or a good healthy respect for the consequences. Having a healthy amount of fear is not the same as losing energy worrying.

If you have a subject that needs to be "worried out," this is a way to do it thoroughly and efficiently. Either way, the goal is to take action sooner or later.

I worry about:

Events _____
Relationships _____
Health _____
Other's Health _____
Money _____
Job _____
Embarrassment _____
Failure _____
Rejection _____
Other _____

Now cross out those categories about which you can do nothing. From those that remain, chose the most important worries and write them below:

My all-time all-star worry	My next important worry	My next important worry	My next important worry

Write as many worries as you need to, using other paper if necessary. Go through the list and ask yourself, Can I do anything about this today? Mark Y for *yes* and N for *no* by each entry. Recopy all the "y's" below:

_____

_____

_____

Next to each worry, write what action you will take today. After you take action on each, write below any that remain unresolved, and what action to take on another day. Copy these onto your calendar, selecting an appropriate day for each. Be careful to not expect too much of yourself.

_____

_____

_____

Now copy all the "N's" below, those that for one reason or another you could not take action on within this day.

_____

_____

_____

Now go through the N list you have written above and ask yourself, Will this get better or worse if I do nothing? Write B for better, S for same, and W for worse.

_____

_____

_____

Copy all the "W's" below.

_____

_____

_____

Consider only the "W's". Assuming that you now have a smaller list, answer in writing each of the questions below for each of the items:

1. Do I want to solve this problem?
2. What am I doing about this right now?
3. What will I need to do about this situation in the near future?
4. Do I need to evaluate my approach?
5. What is the worst that can happen?
6. Is it likely to happen?

7. How about second worst?
8. Can I live with that?
9. Does my thinking about it help the situation?
10. Does my thinking about this problem make it worse?
11. Is there anywhere I can go for help with this problem?
12. What's keeping me from getting help?

Now consider only the items that: 1). you can do something about; and 2). that thinking about can help. Now answer, for each of these:

1. What can I do about this today?
2. What can I do about this tomorrow?
3. What can I do about this next week?
4. What can I do about this next month?
5. What can I do about this next year?

On a calendar write in the appropriate space exactly what you are going to do on which day (at a certain time, if possible) about each problem.

Example: You have decided that only your friend Carl can advise you on this problem. (We'll call it subject z.) Carl is in Africa until April. So write on your calendar: *April 2, phone Carl about subject z*. On April 2, after you have talked to Carl and decided what to do about subject z, mark on your calendar the next date you need to think about this problem.

Do this for each problem. You have now divided up your worries into reasonable groupings, separated those that need action from those that don't need action. Now you can let your calendar remind you of how much attention you need to give to the item. Each time you take action on an item, write what action you took and the results. Then transfer the subject to another date on your calendar, along with the intended action. When it's resolved, discard the subject from your worry list.

Never give any subject on your list energy without taking appropriate action. If you are unsure of the action you plan to take, run it through this set of questions:

This is my decision: I am deciding whether to ____
- If I decide yes, this is what I want to happen:

  _____
- If I decide yes, this is what most likely will happen: _____
- If I decide yes, this is the worst that can happen:

  _____
- If I decide no, this is what I want to happen:

  _____
- If I decide no, this is most likely to happen: ____

  _____
- If I decide no, this is the worst that can happen:

  _____
- What really stands in my way from making this decision? _____

  _____
- What's at stake? _____

  _____
- What am I willing to risk? _____

  _____
- Can I survive looking like a fool? _____

  _____

- If my feelings are hurt, am I strong enough to overcome it? _____

- Can I afford to lose what I have now? _____

- What am I really frightened of? _____

- Is it worth sacrifice of better things if I allow myself the opportunity to fail? _____

- Is it the truth that I choose things as they are now? _____

In six months, look again at your original list of worries. Note which have been resolved and which still need work. Take action and sleep well!

Daring to Fail

Behold the turtle. He only makes progress when he sticks his neck out.

— James Bryant Conant

Only she who attempts the absurd can achieve the impossible.

— Bumper sticker

Fear of failure is a specific kind of fear that often holds

people back from expressing their real potential. Failure is perceived as, at best, embarrassing, and at worst, something from which people are afraid they will have difficulty rallying. Fear is the great inhibitor of change and the checkmate of free-flowing energy.

One of the world's most famous men was labeled by his political enemies "the orangutan from Illinois" before he became one of the most remembered Presidents of the United States. Here is what Abraham Lincoln's record would look like if you were scrutinizing only his defeats:[142]

- 1831 — His business failed.
- 1832 — He was defeated for the legislature.
- 1833 — His business failed again.
- 1838 — He was defeated for Speaker of the House.
- 1840 — He was defeated for Elector.
- 1848 — He was defeated for Congress.
- 1855 — He was defeated for the Senate.
- 1856 — He was defeated for the Vice-Presidential nomination.
- 1858 — He was defeated for the Senate, although his party swept the nation.

If you look hard enough, you can find that many of the world's more interesting achievers have left a trail of "failures" behind them. Lincoln didn't get hung up on his record or he would have quit early and never gone on to greatness. All achievers have a record that isn't completely filled with stunning successes. Let's be careful what we look for — especially in ourselves.

Squeezing Lemons

When life hands you a lemon, make lemonade.
— Anonymous Folk Wisdom

How do we know what a challenge is if there is no risk of failure? How do we find our limits? If we never experience failure, we may be playing it too safe. Since all risks worth taking have the possibility of not working, a failure doesn't have to be viewed as a failure, especially when it's a learning experience. Perhaps it's a guidepost marking the place to take a turn in another direction. Maybe it's a message from yourself to "go for it" and try harder. Risk is an unavoidable part of growth and change, an inevitable part of creative living. Here are ways to approach fear of failure.

Retell Your Story in Glowing Terms When you are stuck in a difficult situation, when life hands you a bouquet of sandburs instead of what you expected, you can work to change how you feel by retelling the story in the best terms you can. If you repeat it often, like an affirmation, it starts to feel true.

Rachel is a highly successful designer with an international reputation. When she spoke to me initially, she talked of the expectations she still carried from her Catholic childhood and of her guilt feelings over her "failure to marry". Although she is still struggling with this issue, the last time we talked she told her story in a different way. Now she spoke of her "decision to stay single, her commitment to her career, her passion for good design." She makes it a point on traditional holidays (previously a low time for her) to drink a toast to her "outrageously successful independence."

If you cannot change the facts as Rachel did, change what they mean to you. Shakespeare had the right idea when he said, "There is no right or wrong, but thinking makes it so."

Name the Problem   How you name your problem reveals much about how you intend to solve it. Which of the following speakers would you be most likely to hire?

"I've been fired."

"I've been canned."

"I'm in between jobs."

"I'm going on to new opportunities."

Learn from It   One way to detach yourself from failure is by viewing it as a lesson: "What a valuable lesson! Guess I learned a lot from it." Failure teaches us things (like how to survive failure). It also teaches us to empathize with others who experience what may be called failure one day, and a stepping-stone to success on another.

State What's Safe   Identify the problem by stating the part of it that is not a problem. Make a list starting with the words "I feel safe . . ." For example, if the fear is of public speaking, write all the parts of it that would not be a problem: I feel safe speaking to four people at once. (Is five too many? Or six?) I feel safe speaking if I am not seen. (Like on radio?) I feel safe speaking if I read the text from a paper. I feel safe speaking if I know my subject. I feel safe speaking if people are asking me questions for which I know the answers. I feel safe speaking if what I have to say helps people.

Look at your list and plan how you can carry these

notions into action. Once you have actually accomplished the "safe" parts, try another portion that is riskier. Action builds confidence!

Inner Advisor   An actress told me that when she wants to call up some extra courage she conjures up a character from inside herself that she has named Adventurous Little Girl. This little friend has a wealth of wisdom about risk-taking, has good instincts for danger, no irrational fears, and embodies the most interesting characteristics of the actress herself. Trusting her is the actress's way of identifying and trusting the strongest part of herself.

Travel Fast   People concerned less with failure than how others will view it have used the "travel fast" approach: Everything is permanently temporary, especially failure. By the time anyone hears about it, it's history. You are off and running on your way to new success.

Land Softly   Give yourself the opportunity to fail by deciding at the outset that risking failure is worth it. Determine in advance that the possibility of failure is the price of success. If you are really stretching to your potential, you will have lots of opportunity to fail and thus be pretty good at it. Failing gracefully is one of the most obvious signs of greatness.

Join Distinguished Company   Failure hurts. How is it possible to risk success? Or failure? It helps to remember that:

- Even Leonardo da Vinci was turned down once in a while.
- Some best-selling manuscripts have been rejected dozens of times before being accepted.
- At least one-half of all contestants in athletic

meets lose. They don't refuse to play the game because of the high risks. It's part of seeking challenge.

- Actors, dancers, and musicians all risk rejection every time they go for an audition. Sometimes they have to take risks just to get an audition.
- You don't always have to win to succeed in life. Likewise, you don't have to receive A's in school in order to know success. Do you know what they call the person who finished last in the medical school class? Doctor.

Taming the Cowardly Lion

I am an old man and I have known many troubles, but most of them never happened.

— Mark Twain

Following are some approaches to fears and worrying. I do not expect you to try them all. Choose the one(s) that is/are best suited to your style and situation.

Examine Your Fear Critically   Is your mental image of the danger realistic? One way to test this is to compare it with that of a respected and seemingly less fearful friend. Would this friend be afraid? Do you respect this friend's judgment.?

Divide and Conquer   Break up your fear into small pieces and tackle them one at a time. If you are afraid of flying, arrange to walk into a plane while it is on the ground. You do not plan to take a trip. You are not really leaving. You do not have a ticket. You have arranged to "just visit" a plane that is not going anywhere, knowing you will walk out of it again. (This is probably easiest to arrange at a flight school, rather than at a commercial airline.)

Then, take another step, like a talking to a pilot or visiting the observation deck of a high building. Try to pinpoint exactly what your fear is. One person who was afraid to fly conquered the fear after she realized her specific fear was that the restroom would not be available in case she became airsick. Another found he'd be fine it he didn't look out the window.

Affirm Away Your Fears   Ann Buran, Midwest coordinator for Omega Seminars, has a list of what she calls "emergency affirmations." While hiking in the mountains of Peru, she found herself in a situation in which she had to cross a narrow ledge, wide enough only for her feet, on the edge of a sheer precipice. She stopped, centered herself into a relaxed pose, visualized herself safely on the other side, and replaced any negative monologue in her head with positive words. "I thoroughly enjoy standing in this beautiful high place and am confident and capable as I walk safely across." She could and she did.

You do not need to eliminate all fears from your life, just bring fear to a level that enhances your life-style. It is our little fears, along with our desires, that make us unique and interesting.

Explore Your Feelings   Learn more about your fears by completing the following sentences: What I really am afraid of is _____

Now WordSpin your answer. Write what you have learned here. _____

_____

Thought Replacements for Risk-taking and Fears

- So what? Life is a game. It's only a game.
- I trust myself.
- I fearlessly accept today. Today is mine!
- I have courage.
- Go in peace.
- Stop! This is not the truth. The truth is . . . .
- Be Not Afraid. (Familiar words seen on a sign in the office of Mayor Koch of New York City)
- It doesn't look life-threatening and anything else is unimportant. (From a financial executive who calmly and fearlessly invests millions daily)
- I am ferocious. (This is used by women who ride New York subways, on the premise that if you don't look or feel like a victim you are less likely to be victimized.)

Affirmations for Fears and Worries

- Whatever challenge I meet today I can handle successfully.
- "God's in heaven and all's right with the world."
  —Browning
- I am free of irrational fears others have taught me.
- I trust myself.

Step 12. Keeping Energy Moving

Energy is nothing if it's not moving. The superachievers and effective energists interviewed in all parts of the country have one thing in common — they keep their energy moving in consciously chosen directions. Some have used their energy to change their physical surroundings; others, their social, spiritual, or emotional environments. Some have consciously turned inward for answers that created changes in their outside world. Some directed their energy outward, energized others, and, subsequently, themselves.

The way your energy flows is determined largely by how you decide to direct it. By taking it in, allowing it to flow through you, then giving it away, you seem to grow in energy capacity. Energy going out for positive ends energizes the sender anew. When you put your energy behind what you truly love, you are unstoppable.

When free-flowing energy moves you in a positive direction, it's like a golden path in front of you. It's "following the joy."[143] When the energy feels good, like joy, the work is good. That's how you know when to continue.

In this concluding section we'll explore the lives of several people who have developed diverse and satisfying energy styles.

To Rest Is to Rust (or, How to Inherit Good Genes)

Energetic George Montague Eberhardt, who was born in 1904, says he never exercises. He says he doesn't believe in exercise, or doing anything in particular for longevity. He believes it's enough to just keep breathing. I should have suspected something fishy about this when he told me he takes phone calls only between seven and seven-thirty in the morning.

George dropped out of college to become a messenger at Western Electric. Later he worked at Bell Laboratories in research and development, where he helped pioneer intercontinental radio communications, a career that took him all over the Western hemisphere. He retired from Bell in 1966 after forty-four years of employment.

Then George started a second career as Director of Audio Facilities at Drew University. He had held this post for seventeen years when I interviewed him.

George is passionate about excellent sound reproduction. He can turn a classroom into a quality sound studio, install sound systems for theater productions and rock concerts, and repair everything audio that breaks down.

His cluttered laboratory looks like a sorcerer's workshop. For the last four years he has accompanied the college choir on its annual tour to record the concerts. Traveling with a busload of college students (to Canada in 1985) is not how everyone would choose to spend a spring vacation, but George says he is energized by the young people. (This is a good thing, since he has also been known to take them roller skating.)

What he said was true: George Eberhardt never *deliberately* sets out to do any activity just for exercise. Instead, from his youth on, action was his habit and physical activity was an integral part of his daily routine. His activities in his adult life have included twenty-one different sports, including fencing and high jumping. (He didn't say when he retired from that.) His résumé lists as many as twenty-seven avocations, including house design and construction, farm chores, and volunteer fireman.

In addition to his work at Drew, George has several sideline businesses, including a tennis court maintenance service and a professional audio transfer and recording business. He still teaches tennis.

With an active life like this, who needs exercise? I felt exercised just following George Eberhardt around. He works outdoors several days a week, maintaining clay tennis courts. Tennis, which he has played regularly since he was sixteen, provides fresh air and exercise. When he is on campus, reaching, bending, climbing ladders, and hanging cables, the work encourages muscle and joint flexibility. Transporting heavy recorders and speakers around involves a lot of weight-lifting. Carrying the equipment up steps in campus buildings is heavy aerobic activity. When I told him he practices a total exercise program, complete with weight-lifting and sustained aerobic activity, he laughed. "It's just good genes," he says. "I was astute in my choice of parents." Then he told me an outrageous story about being descended from the fighting Montague family of *Romeo and Juliet* fame.

George will concede that moving a lot was a tradition in his family. "My grandfather said, 'To rest is to rust.' I was always surrounded by people who were active. I grew up thinking this was the way of life, so like a gyroscope, I just wind up." He circles his finger in the air to illustrate his point.

Researchers and gerontologists agree with George that heredity is a factor, but it is not the whole picture. Knowing your heredity and working with it can considerably alter your pattern of health. If you know that heart disease runs in your family, for example, you can take steps to remove yourself from the high-risk group. According to the National Center for Health Statistics in Washington, D.C., simply by doing the things that help one avoid heart disease, you can add as much as fifteen years to your life!

If you want to live long and energetically, start exercising early. With an eye toward a long and active life, you might consider emulating George in other ways:

- Be well nourished.
- Having stimulating social contacts (George boasts several generations of coeds who adoringly adopted him as "Grandpa.")
- Do what you love. Have many interests and stay alive intellectually.
- Have strong family connections. (George has a

large and affectionate family circle — ten grandchildren and "at least four great-grandchildren").

- Be curious. (George says, "I'm curious about
  everything. I don't climb a mountain just because
  it's there, but because I want to know what's
  on the other side.)

- Laugh. (George has a rousing sense of humor.
  He occasionally writes a humor column for the
  campus newspaper.)

George likes to play with words, especially when it
means tripping up faculty members at the college. If someone asks him how many "kids" he has, George, always
excruciatingly accurate, replies, "None. I'm not an old
goat!"

I didn't want to fall into the trap, so I asked him how
many children he had. "I didn't actually have any of the
children myself," he said. "But my first wife produced
two children. My second wife had five. My third wife
had none. In fact, I don't have a third wife. I told my
second wife when she was sixty — that was two years
ago — that I was going to trade her in for two thirties."
He wouldn't tell me what Mrs. Eberhardt's reaction was,
or how he got the scar on his chest, except to say that
it was from a high-heeled shoe.

Remember the phrase from the beginning of the book
— "What you love grows?" George is a master at following
his interests and turning them into exciting careers and
avocations.

Do you experience the flow of energy available to you
by doing the things you love? To check, WordSpin the
phrase with which you complete this sentence: When I'm

really honest with myself, the activity I'm most passionate about is _____.

Complete the exercise with a short paragraph, beginning, What I learned was _____
_____
_____.

What did you learn? Are you putting your energy behind your interests? If not, take action.

Maggie Reinventing Herself

Maggie picked me up in her snappy little yellow convertible, with the top down at five o'clock on a chilly morning, for a drive from New Jersey to Martha's Vineyard to visit a mutual friend. I was up and ready, but unprepared for sunny, energetic Maggie. Maggie is one of those rare women whose appearance is enhanced by early hours and the windblown look. I had known Maggie for several years as a fast-paced and stylish executive, trainer, and consultant, a bold adventurer who was getting her pilot's license, a divorced mother of two grown children. On the way to the island she told me about her personal transformation from Maggie the "energetic frenetic," as she described herself, to Maggie now at peace with the process of reinventing herself.

"I have more energy now than I have ever had. I think it's because I have reached a state in which I am not struggling so much. My energy is being used productively, not being dissipated by excessive concerns and worries. With the achievement of this peace has come a sense of knowing about myself, so this is also a result of self-mastery. To me, self-mastery was a term that I never understood and never had any idea that I could have it, but I wanted it. I watched people around me, thinking that they must have it, so I was going after what I thought they had."

Maggie says she was born with high energy. She claims that having high energy, if it is not tempered by discipline and order, is exhausting, which is why she was so determined to achieve some control over it. She was pleased to learn that she did not have to give up her peppy pace to do this, that achieving peace of mind while maintaining an active life-style *is* possible. Maggie spent a lot of time and energy getting control of her life. She went about the search for inner peace the same way she went about everything else in her life: furiously. She started with a meditation class, and if anyone could meditate with fury, Maggie did. This experience opened her mind to the paths for self-change. She went on from there to other kinds of self-development seminars, eventually becoming a trainer herself.

"The EST training gave me a sense of my own power to create.[144] Studying and teaching DMA gave me the tools to use that power and energy so that I could create what I wanted.[145] I learned that if I accepted certain circumstances and then noticed that I didn't particularly care for the circumstances I could choose to take a new direction. That's very empowering. Also, I'm in the right work — work that's a good expression of me. That's energizing.

"I'm not wasting my energy on stress. I've come to terms with not having life go perfectly all the time. I'm accepting life for the moment — living life in the now. Living in the moment for me is very peaceful. I love not worrying! Worrying is the concern that you won't be able to handle or cope with life satisfactorily, and I'm confident that I can and that I do."

Maggie didn't always have her life so well under control. In the process of reinventing herself, Maggie has gone through many changes. When she was young, she rebelled against her orderly, controlling family. "I admired discipline, but I refused to be disciplined because I wanted to be the free spirit. When I was younger, I wouldn't even write out a list, no matter what, because I thought it would be conforming to the way that most people did things. I would somehow get by — by the seat of my pants, usually. It's funny, but it was very vitalizing in a way, because I was totally living the way I wanted to live, and that felt very good. It was momentarily satisfying because I could say, See? I did it anyway! I'm not doing it the way somebody else told me to do it. I'm doing it my way. But it wasn't particularly rewarding. So now I choose to be orderly, and it feels wonderful, being orderly because I choose it, rather than having somebody else tell me that was the way to do things."

Maggie wanted order in her life, but she had to choose to be free first. When this was an accomplished fact, she chose to be orderly and disciplined. She found that this enhanced her productivity and satisfaction.

Like any truly creative act, real originality must emerge after a period of letting go, and this may feel like undirected chaos. For Maggie, the first key to letting go was her introduction to meditation. For some people this first letting-go of the internal controls occurs in an almost religious moment. What Maggie found in her determined pursuit of inner peace was that by letting go, she was able to free herself enough to find a direction that was truly her own.

"I am still going in the direction that I have chosen, but now I have let go of the controls. It's like sailing. I am not going to try to control the winds, but I can adjust the sail and rudder for the direction that the wind is blowing. I still have my target, so I am controlling under the circumstances. In this sense I feel I am very much in control.

"An example of this is when a man I was dating decided to break up (with me). I knew that I had precipitated the breakup, but it didn't make it any easier to accept. We were flying back in a single-engine plane at night from a wonderful dinner. He was going through all these weak excuses about why we probably shouldn't date steadily, and I was so upset that I was absolutely ready to jump out of the airplane. What I was upset about was not being able to control our relationship. I thought I was going to go nuts. I made the decision then that I was going to let go of feeling that I had to have everything, moment to moment, exactly as I wanted it. In my rational moments I realize that you cannot control somebody else's life. You cannot control the moment. The moment is the moment. To accept the moment is being in control. Then you can choose what you want the next moment. If I had done that on the airplane that night, rather than spending my energy trying to figure out how to get back in control of the relationship, and how to get him to want me again [poor pitiful me, he chose the twenty-nine-year-old over me] . . . if I had looked at the moment with acceptance and said, 'This is the way it is' and then looked to see what I wanted, I would have been back in control, not of his life, but of mine. I was still trying to manipulate the moment, having it be the way that it wasn't, rather than let it be the way that it was.

"Trying to control is so draining. Now I have a sense of peace. I am not trying all the time to adjust to my situation. Now it's an acceptance of the situation. It's the lack of needing to manipulate circumstances anymore. I accept the way it is."

People who have a sense of control in their lives are more confident, satisfied, and tend to experience events as an outgrowth of their own actions, rather than as demons that creep up to overwhelm them unprepared. Fearless and bold actions lead to more fearless and bold actions, which encourage a more interesting and energetic life. Yet being too controlling brings its own problems, as Maggie described. It's like sailing or riding a horse. The wind and the horse must be respected, too.

These are the steps Maggie experienced in the process of reinventing herself:

Loving Herself   Being true to herself in her choices. She needed to be free to choose disciplined and orderly behavior for herself, not because her family wanted this for her but because she wanted it.

Mastering the Tools   In Maggie's case, meditation was the key that led to her attending other self-development seminars. She eventually became a leader in this and made it her career. Others will seek other paths, but the road that creates real change always begins with an inside journey.

Remaining Flexible and Accepting Change   Each

change is part of the process, not the end in itself. Learning to read life's signals in a positive way allows the opportunity to choose again. Coming up against an obstacle is not a failure but a signal that energy is not flowing. Maggie has no fear of decisions, because she has the opportunity to right the course later.

Taking Control   For Maggie, this meant assessing her own talents, skills, needs, and goals, assuming responsibility for them and directing her energy in productive ways.

Letting Go of the Controls   Having the confidence that the process she had set into motion would take care of itself, she was able to quit worrying and manipulating. Letting go allows for the unexpected: happy accidents, serendipitous happenings. It allows for real relationships.

Letting Love Energy Flow   Are you sailing with or against the wind? Life never occurs in straight lines so, as Maggie said, we always have another choice, another zig or another zag to change direction if we wish, but always guided by our course direction.

Self-Love and Independence

I don't want to let Maggie's first definition of *Love* pass by without further explanation. In the section called "What You Love Grows," I used the word *love* to mean "having a consuming interest in" or "being passionately enthusiastic about" something. Loving our world, children, nature, our life in general, or a specific part of it — like our interests, work, or hobbies — can be a great energizer. This kind of "passion" (when it's not ego-based or an obsession) moves us closer to our goals and helps us to feel good about ourselves. Anything that enhances our self-esteem also enhances our ability to "love" in the other senses of the word.

Love is basic for a satisfying and energized life. I don't mean to limit this to love between two people, which seems to be what many think of first when they hear the word *love*. Unconditional love doesn't have that limitation; it can come from many sources. The best source is within yourself. This kind of love heals bruises and bridges our separateness and is not limited to one other person.

Maggie found that letting go of the need to control was letting go of her need to be attached to someone else's energy, a condition she had earlier described as "love."

Maggie's definition of love was based upon dependence. It wasn't love, but need. Need gets in the way of love. Needy love is an example of energy that is not flowing, or flowing all in one direction. When Maggie said she was ready to jump out of the plane because she couldn't manipulate this man into wanting her, she was illustrating the kind of problem that needy love causes. Mistaking neediness for love, Maggie had gotten her energy temporarily stuck in someone else's energy field. Fortunately, she had the tools with which to disentangle herself.

Getting stuck in someone else's energy field because it feels good is a common problem, especially for women. Loving yourself first is the way out of this situation. Strong and mature love can occur only between two mutually independent people secure in self-love. This kind of interdependence preserves the integrity and individuality of both parties. It includes the freedom to flow with one's own energy and to make rational and energizing decisions.[146]

This kind of strong love based on self-esteem respects the self, while recognizing and accepting and respecting the total person who is the object of that love. This isn't easy. Often called "unconditional love," it means loving, accepting, respecting the other without trying to remodel that person into one's own image. When love is unconditional, the person who is the object of that love is allowed to grow in his or her own direction. Loving a person who is growing and changing in directions apart from our own invites conflict, but that, too, encourages healthy growth. To insulate one's self from this kind of pain is to refuse to grow and results not in unconditional love, but in unending boredom.

I like what the sage Tagore said: "Let my love, like sunlight, surround you and yet give you illumined freedom."[147]

Getting stuck in another's energy field doesn't happen only in romantic situations. Becoming addicted to another, more powerful person's energy field is what happens in cults when people get stuck in "guru trips," following charismatic leaders.

The groupies are sensitive enough to recognize the presence of a stronger energy conduit. What they don't realize is that they could become conduits for this energy on their own and still remain effective, functioning individuals. Becoming spiritually and intellectually imprisoned in "secondhand" energy is a weak, dependent state and an ineffectual way of using energy. These leaders may actually be conduits for a higher form of energy or they may be simply using their energy more effectively than most of us. Either way, it is a misuse of this power to take advantage of others, as is happening in various cults.

Humans have a need to be part of a circle. Energists are strong hardy people who can remain individualistic within a functioning social system. Energists can lean and be leaned upon. This is not weakness, but a way to stay strong and independent. Holding ourselves separate from others takes energy. Separateness itself can make us more susceptible to disease. People with strong ties to others are healthier, live longer, have fewer health problems, and endure stressful events more easily, researchers find.[148] Women undergoing pregnancy with high stress levels but strong social ties had fewer complications than similar women who had no supportive network.[149]

Individualism isn't selfishness and it isn't incompatible with being a good group player. It's dancing in the center of your own circle, a much more rewarding position than being on the periphery of another's turf.

By loving yourself first you remain free and personally powerful. People who exhibit what is called star quality, charm, personal magnetism, and charisma probably were not born this way. This mystical glow can be learned and it starts with cherishing number one — yourself.

Loving yourself is a revolutionary act — revolutionary in the true sense: It can change things in yourself and others. We started out by saying that "What you love grows." When you love yourself, your energy flows, your influence grows. People look to you for guidance and example. The world that you perceive becomes perceived by others, so if you are going to become energized and powerful, let it be love energy that propels you.

Visualizing Your Energetic Self

Can you visualize yourself vital, energetic, *fully* alive? Can you stretch your imagination to include your optimal self? Can you create a very clear and detailed picture, as if you are watching a movie of yourself? This exercise will guide you. (This will work best if you record this on to a tape for playback. You may want to change the words into the first person — that is, substitute the word "I" for the word "You.")

Relax, using one of the methods previously discussed. Keep the inner image positive, clear, and vivid. Use the questions only to help yourself make your visualization stronger. *Do not attempt to actively answer the questions in words. Let the questions guide your imaging. Allow the images to float in and out. Accept what comes without judgment.*

1. Visualize yourself in a pleasant situation, feeling vital and energized. Keep the image light and positive.
2. How does this energetic self look?
3. What is this energetic self doing?
4. What is this energetic self wearing?
5. What is the environment?
6. Is this energetic self playing or working?

7. Are other people present?
8. Can you find something in this image to admire?
9. Notice your enjoyment of this activity.
10. *Feel* the enjoyment.
11. Repeat to yourself one or more of the following:
    - I enjoy being alive and energetic.
    - I enjoy being totally healthy and effective in every way.
    - I enjoy my active life-style.
    - I deserve to be a healthy, vital, and energetic person. This health, vitality, and energy comes to me and flows through me for the highest good of all.

Come back as soon as your vision fades or your mind wanders. Treat this process like a game and keep it light and easy. Focusing upon the enjoyment of the image, either verbally or as part of your visual image, makes your visualization more powerful. Repeat this visualization as often as you wish.

Collecting Energizing People

As you become more energized, other energists will seek you out. People find energetic people attractive, but attracting people is only one step to creating your own support system. Such networks must be nurtured and loved.

In a very real sense, you create your friends and what they mean to you. They do not magically become the personnel in your life. It takes time and attention to build a network of supportive friends. The returns are very much worth the investment.

The way you direct your energy, the accumulation of small and large decisions, and your choice of personal interests encourages some friends and discourages others. Cumulatively, these acts determine the cast of characters in your life. It may happen unconsciously, but just as certainly as if you were a stage director, you mold and shape these "actors" in your life story. When you say, I really like it when you ———, you are likely to set up a pattern for that behavior to be repeated. When you give encouragement you are setting up energy patterns in another person's life. When you care about a friend enough to recommend or loan a book, or to phone just to say hello, you set the stage for a future contact with this person, drawing this person into a larger role in your life.

If you give your friends loving attention, they will become fruitful and multiply. If you let them, they will darken your door and tie up your phone. This may be just what you want. Or, like exercise, health food and raising puppies, you can get too much of any good thing. If you love yourself first, you will find the balance.

The Hug List
Make a list of all the people you like to hug. Add the people you would like be hugged by. Add any other person you would hug if you had the opportunity or the nerve.

HUGGABLE PEOPLE	HOW LONG SINCE YOU LAST TALKED?
1.	_____
2.	_____
3.	_____
4.	_____
5.	_____
6.	_____
7.	_____

(You may need more space.)

Now look at your list and see what you can do about it. Write a letter? Phone someone? Just give someone a big hug?

Group Energy

You can gain energy from like-minded people. There are religious groups, parenting groups, music groups, psychic groups, exercise groups, meditation groups. There are groups to promote intercultural understanding, groups to help people end their addictions, groups to help people overcome grief, groups for all kinds of personal development.

Sometimes when people come together in a group with common values and the same focus, whether at a football game, in a religious service, or at a political rally, something happens, something that has to do with the manifestation of energy. We can't explain exactly what happens, but witnesses attest that *something* happens, something that can't be measured by our available instruments. Sometimes people call it spirit (as in school spirit) or charisma.

The Rev. Robert Corin Morris, both in his capacity as a clergyperson and as the director of the interdenominational Interweave Center, spends a lot of time with groups. He says, "To people who are energy aware, it's as if the group is creating a common group energy field. One of the things that's necessary for this phenomenon to occur is that the whole group be willing to flow with it, not fight what is happening and not bring in conflicts or disagreements."[150]

Reverend Morris recalls a dramatic incident when this happened. "A woman was being ordained and about twenty ministers were standing around with their hands on her head for almost ten minutes because the minister who was leading the pastoral prayer for ordination went on at some length. For the first two or three minutes it was like a normal church service. Then I became aware of heat and electricity in the group, then a sort of common pulsebeat, and the whole group began moving. It was like a throbbing light.

"I thought, 'This is very interesting,' but I really assumed that it was my own private perception, until after the ordination part was over. The moderator for the state in which the ordination took place seemed to be genuinely shaken. He said, 'I have these prepared remarks, but I really can't say them, because I've never experienced anything like that before in my life, and I don't even know what it was.' Then the moderator went on to describe the experience that I had had in very much the same terms. At the reception, many people described it the same way. The most common description of it was light, heat, warmth, and pulsebeat and the sensation that we were all one great pulsing heart."

When Reverend Morris emphasizes that this energy

is spirit with the small "s," he is making an important differentiation. He is saying that when people get together, they sometimes form an energy field. (Their brain waves or heartbeats may begin to synchronize.) He is not saying that this phenomenon necessarily has any supernatural power or meaning. It simply may be a yet unexplained property of human energy.

While this phenomenon is more readily recognized when it happens in large groups, this energy exchange happens on some level whenever people meet. Have you noticed that you can *almost see* sparks between people who are in love? That people who are sexually attracted to each other seem to be joined by invisible cables that draw them together? Sometimes you meet someone to whom you feel instantly attracted. Whether male or female, same sex, romantically involved, or just friends, this person seems to energize and bring out the best in you. Our language has no words for this, only colloquialisms derived from physics, such as "on the same wave length."

Sometimes the opposite happens. You introduce two people who have everything in common, including their antique harmonica collections, and everything stops cold. It's dislike-at-first-sight, a perfect example of energy not moving.

Tuning in to these social situations can have some practical applications. Good salespeople sense the energy flow and know when to push and when to back off. Actors tune in to the audience's energy to create an exciting performance. Parents can often feel their children's moods. A real estate investor told me he can "smell" a good buy.

Although it is rarely recognized as such, many important decisions are made on intuitive knowledge, which is at least in part the "feel" of the energy flow. One way to know if a path is right is to determine whether energy feels freely flowing. If it's not, it's trying to tell you something, although signals like this are not always clear. "I just *knew* it was the thing to do!" expresses this kind of intuitive response. When the energy feels stuck, or is blocked and you feel unable to take action, it's likely something is not working. It's time to try a new direction.[151]

Gaining Energy by Giving Energy

When Janice Howard[152] was a young graduate student, she went to Nicaragua (then under the rule of Anastasio Somoza) to help design a new psychiatric facility. The conditions there would have been enough to frighten off the faint of heart. Criminals were kept in the same building as people who were depressed or suffering from epilepsy. Some people were kept naked in cages. Janice didn't retreat, but stayed to help the architect design a more appropriate and humane facility.

While in Nicaragua, Janice was asked to transform a donated house in a leper colony into a school for the lepers' children. Although no funds were appropriated for this project, Janice was aware of the real and urgent need to provide a place for these children away from their homes because this gave them their only chance to avoid contracting the disease.

As I interviewed Janice, while watching the night lights of beautiful San Diego harbor, we seemed so far from leprosy, jungles, and dictators. Janice told me her story. "I went out to the leper colony the first day with the social worker, a very classy woman. I don't know how to describe my reaction. Leprosy looks so grotesque. The people's faces are all eaten up and mangled — it's not a nice sight. When one of the worst-looking of the colony residents came up and gave the social worker a big hug and a kiss, I thought, 'Gosh! If that man touches me, I'll just die! I don't know what I'm going to do!'

"Then we went to talk to one of the doctors. I said, 'I want to know — am I going to get this? Because I'm not sure that this is where I want to be.'

"He said, 'Well, I'm here, and I haven't gotten it.' He told me that it is only through prolonged contact that you get the disease."

In spite of Janice's fear, the challenge felt right. "We had to go around to different businesses to get donations for materials, for paint, lumber, nails, for tile — for anything we used. Probably because we were young and foolish American women who didn't know any better, they gave us the donations that we needed. A couple of architectural students and a couple from the Peace Corps helped. We just tore the place apart and remodeled it.

"The work energized me! I was never so driven. I'm a high-energy person, but I'm not a morning person. Not at all. In Nicaragua, that was the one time that I would be awake, just like a shot at six-thirty in the morning. I would be out of the house by seven. My fear was there but what I was doing seemed so important at the time that I didn't let it stop me.

"I think, yes, in the back of my mind for the whole time I worked there, I wondered if I would get leprosy.

Part of me was still afraid but it's so devastating to see those children. If nobody did anything, they'd end up just like their parents.

"Many of the residents of the colony were young, in their twenties. They have no work, nothing to do all day, and they wanted to help with the building. One young man came over and asked me if he could help with the sawing. I looked at him and saw that he didn't have any fingers. I didn't want to be mean, so I said, 'That's very nice of you to offer, but that's okay, we're doing okay.'

"'No,' he said. 'I want to help.'

"I said, 'Can you saw this board for me?'

"He had his own saw, an old rusty saw. He went to the kitchen and got a bowl of vegetable oil and greased that thing and in three minutes flat he had that board cut and wanted to know what else he could do. After he broke the ice, the other men helped us, too. Their contribution was so valuable, and they felt such a sense of accomplishment.

"When the house was done we built a jungle gym, very simple — all we had was plywood and two-by-fours. We got someone to donate some rope and we strung that up. It was the first time that these little kids ever had anything like that.

"At the grand opening the people from the leper colony were invited for punch and cookies. One of the donations we had gotten was an aquarium. The older people had not seen fish. They stared at the fish tank for hours. We take so much for granted. The last I heard, the child-care center was still operating."

Janice was energized by the work that needed to be done. It gave her the courage to overcome her fears and take the risk that the work demanded. In Nicaragua she truly experienced what is meant by "keeping energy moving," which has become a habit with Janice and is a continuing source of courage for her as well. A few years ago, when her partner withdrew at the last minute from starting an interior design company with her, Janice believed in herself enough to go ahead on her own. Now she is president of J. Howard Associates, the San Diego interior design firm she founded. Her business is expanding to include a large staff and clients from all over the country.

Reaching Out: Creating a Friendly World

When Albert Einstein was asked, "What do you find to be the most important question of our time?," he surprised the questioner by replying, "Is the universe friendly?"

In every dimension, cosmically or in our own neighborhoods, it takes a lot of energy to live in a hostile world. To make our world friendlier is an inside job — inside ourselves. But inner work doesn't exclude outer action. That's needed as well. Having our inner house in order first makes our outer work more effective.

None of us sees the world in exactly the same way. Instead, we view it through a kind of "telescope" based upon our own world view. We filter new facts through this telescope, most of the time keeping only those that fit our habitual way of thinking. Those with which we don't agree we let slide away from us.

In this way, each of us lives in a world we have created:

the accumulation of our thoughts, fears, desires, choices, beliefs. Having made our world, we can change it.

- By trusting ourselves, we come to trust others.
- By loving ourselves, we can love others.
- By being at peace with ourselves, we can be at peace with others.
- By reaching out, by passionately loving something outside ourselves, we are giving our energy away. Doing so, we create space for more energy to flow into ourselves. Keeping our energy moving gives us more energy.

Jill Jackson Miller loved to write songs. She and her late husband, Sy Miller, wrote one in 1955 that was unlike any of their others. When they finished it, Jill said, "Wonder if anybody will like this. It's a very odd song."

Jill and Sy's song. "Let There Be Peace on Earth and Let It Begin with Me," became one of the most moving and influential ever written. With it they captured the aspirations of the world. This song has energized millions to think about what they can personally do to promote peace.[153] Jill and Sy followed what they loved. Writing songs was the right focus for their energy.

What direction have you chosen for your energy? Many have chosen to work toward creating a friendly earth as a target for their personal energy. Robert Muller, Assistant Secretary General of the United Nations, suggests networking as the way for people to make significant global changes. Great networkers like Gandhi, Jesus, and Martin Luther King, Jr., writes Muller, "have transcended races, nations, and groups and networked at the all-human level, linking the heavens and the earth and showing us our prodigious worth and journey in the universe."[154]

Muller suggests that we do not have to be great net-workers or travel long distances to accomplish great things. Jill and Sy did what they knew how to do and they didn't have to travel any farther than their piano to do it.

Many who are unwilling simply to feel apathetic or depressed about the state of the world have become em-powered by reaching directly to the less fortunate. One of my friends with many children and many problems spends an occasional morning in an inner-city soup kitchen and returns home bouncing with new energy. The Sister City and Friendship City projects (in which U.S. munic-ipalities adopt a city or town in a needy country) offer ways to become involved in people-to-people diplomacy without leaving home. Sending pencils and paper to a school in a jungle or dispatching thermometers and peni-cillin to an orphanage in a country torn by civil strife are only a few of the many ways that "armchair heroes" leave their mark on the world. Opportunities to create a friendlier world appear to us daily. We need only to open ourselves to these possibilities. Giving our talents, energy, and resources multiplies our energy.

Remember our original premise, "What you love grows"? Pierre Teihard de Chardin wrote, "The only hope for survival is the energy of love . . . It can only happen if you believe in it."[155]

Maybe this is a possible idea. Important things have happened when vast numbers of people change their minds just a little. We are all "in process" — as creators of ourselves and our collective future. How we direct our creative energies determines what we will create individually and collectively. People with a strong center of well-directed love energy transform those around them.

We must not underestimate the power of our own energy. You and I are part of a great ever-moving energy shift. When someone moves, everyone else moves over a bit, however imperceptibly. The way that you decide to move moves others. You may be "The 100th Monkey" — the one who makes the difference.[156]

The power in this idealistic-sounding strategy is borne out in public relations theory. Research from Everett Rogers says that when 5% of a society accepts a new idea, it is embedded in its population. After 20% of the population adopts an idea, it is virtually unstoppable.[157] Only 20%! What if 20% decided to put energy into a positive future? Only 20%! Doesn't knowing this make you feel powerful?

Do you have love energy to give? You don't need to go anywhere or be appointed to any special commissions. Love energy is powerful and it's contagious. Love what is sacred to you: the earth, life, love, relationships, art, self-expression. Visualize a future in which what you hold sacred continues to survive. Put your energy into it. Talk it up. Think globally, act locally. Join with other energists of like mind. Whatever you do is the right thing to do. Wherever you are is the right place to do it. Whatever you love is the place to find the give-and-take of energy flow. Keep the energy moving. Follow what you love and people will follow you.

Loving intensely and passionately connects us and makes our personal worlds friendlier because the reverberations of moving love energy are infinite. Reaching out of ourselves, giving our energy away, energizes us as well.

> Love all God's creation, the whole world and every grain of sand in it. Love every leaf, every ray of God's light. Love the animals, love the plants, love everything. If you love everything you will perceive the divine mystery in things. Once you perceive it, you will comprehend it better every day. And you will come at last to love the whole world with an all-embracing love.
>
> — Fyodor Dostoevsky

Notes

1. Gallup Poll for *American Health Magazine* (March 1985), p. 42.
2. John H. Griest, M.D., and colleagues, *Comprehensive Psychiatry* (January/February 1979).
3. Jane E. Brody, "Moderate Level of Exercise Brings Life-Saving Benefits," *The New York Times* (April 9, 1986), p. C1.
4. Ibid.
5. Richard D. Lyons, "Mild Exercise Helps Prolong Life," *The New York Times* (July 27, 1984), p. B7.
6. Jane E. Brody, ". . . Life-Saving Benefits," *The New York Times* (April 9, 1986), p. C1.
7. Ralph S. Paffenbarger, Jr., M.D. et al, "Physical Activity, All-Cause Mortality, and Longevity of College Alumni," *The New England Journal of Medicine*, vol. 314, no. 10 (March 6, 1986), p. 605-612.
8. Neil McAleer, *The Body Almanac* (New York: Doubleday, 1985).
9. Dr. Marcus Bach, Ph.D., "The Power of Total Living," *Science of Mind Magazine*, (June 1982), p. 11.
10. ———, "Lifetime/Exercise," *The Journal of the American Medical Association*, (September 1982).

11. Some of the ideas in this section were developed in conversations with Professor Wilma Gilkey, M.S., instructor in physical education, Middlesex, (N.J.) College, January 25, 1986.

12. Covert Bailey, *Fit or Fat?* (Boston: Houghton Mifflin Company, 1978), p. 105.

13. Ibid.

14. I'm grateful to my hatha yoga teachers: Swami Rama, Judy Freedman, Larry Xavier, and Diana Wolfe.

15. Sandra Blakeslee, "Runners Warned of Mental Danger," *The New York Times* (August 28, 1985).

16. Daniel Goleman, "Staying Up," *Psychology Today*, (March 1982), p. 31.

17. Thomas Coates, Ph.D et al., *Sleep*, vol. 6, no. 2 (April 1983), Reported in *Healthline* (October 1983) p. 19.

18. Constantin R. Soldatos et al, "Cigarette Smoking," *Science*, vol. 207, (February 1980), pp. 551-2.

19. Carl E. Thoresen, Ph.D., "Disturbed Sleep: Taming the Gentle Tyrant," *Healthline*, vol. 2, no. 10 (October 1983), p. 1.

20. Daniel Goleman, Ph.D., "Why Did the Caveman Sleep?", *Psychology Today*, (March 1982), p. 30.

21. Dina Ingber, "Is Sleep a Waste of Time?," *Science Digest*, (April 1984), p. 84.

22. Loretta Lewis, M.A., M.S.W., psychotherapist and adjunct professor at New York University; interview with author, Spring Lake, NJ, July 1985.

23. (Shivarpita), Joan Harrigan, Ph.D. "The Effects of Hatha Yoga Postures and Breathing," *Research Bulletin*, (Honesdale, PA: The Himalayan International Institute, Eleanor N. Dana Laboratory, 1981) vol. 3, nos. 3 and 4, p. 4-5.

24. Some ideas in this section were developed during conversations with wellness educator Janet Harris Ford, M.S., Bacteriology and Public Health.

25. John Noble Wilford, "2 Americans Win Nobel Medicine Prize," *The New York Times* (October 15, 1985), p. A1.

26. William Castelli, M.D., telephone interview with author, January 17, 1986.

27. William Castelli, M.D., provided this information.

28. *The Journal of the American Medical Association* vol. 246 No. 6, (July 2, 1982), p. 640.

29. Daniel W. Cramer, M.D., Sc.D. *Obstetrics and Gynecology* vol. 63 (June 1984), p. 833.

30. Ibid.

31. *The American Journal of Clinical Nutrition* (June 3, 1972).

32. *The Journal of Human Nutrition* vol. 35, no. 6.

33. Jane E. Brody, "New Research on the Vegetarian Diet . . ." *The New York Times* (October 12, 1983), p. C7.

34. *American Journal of Epidemiology* (May 1984).

35. Framingham Heart Study, *The New York Times*, Jan. 8, 1985.

36. William Castelli, M.D., telephone interview with author, January 17, 1986.

37. Rudolph Ballentine, M.D., *Diet and Nutrition* (Honesdale, PA: Himalayan International Institute, 1978), p. 107.

38. Oliver Alabaster, M.D., *What You Can Do to Prevent Cancer*, (New York: Simon and Schuster, 1985), p. 13.

39. Mary Winston, Ed.D., senior science administrator of the American Heart Association, telephone interview with author, January 24, 1986.

40. Jane E. Brody, "Monounsaturated Fats, like Olive Oils . . ." *The New York Times*, (April 29, 1985).

41. Scott M. Grundy, M.D., Ph.D., "Monounsaturated Fatty Acids . . ." *The New England Journal of Medicine*, vol. 314, 12, 1986), pp. 745-48.

42. "Name That Fast Food," *The New York Times* (December 17, 1985), p. A26.

43. Michael F. Jacobson, "Let People Know What They're Eating," *The New York Times* (January 12, 1986).

44. Kathy Pratt, M.S., R.D.; telephone conversation with author, July 7, 1986.

45. A. A. Qureshi, Ph.D., and W. C. Burger, Ph.D.; interview with author, Madison, WI, October 10, 1985.

46. Bud Herron, The *Los Angeles Times Syndicate*, (October 1985).

47. A. A. Qureshi, Ph.D., and W. C. Burger, Ph.D.; interview with author, Madison, WI, October 10, 1985.

48. Oliver Alabaster, M.D., *What You Can Do to Prevent Cancer* (New York: Simon and Schuster, 1985), p. 126.

49. Martin Lipkin M.D. and Harold Newmark, M.S., "Effect of Added Dietary Calcium", *The New England Journal of Medicine*, vol. 313, no. 22 (November 1985), p. 1381.

294

50. *Vegetarian Times*, Suite 921, 41 E. 42nd Street, New York, NY 10017.

51. "From Tofu to Twinkies: What *New Age Journal* Readers Really Eat." *New Age Journal*, (January 1984).

52. Morris Notelovitz, M.D. and Marsha Ware, *Stand Tall!: Every Woman's Guide to Preventing Osteoporosis* (Toronto: Bantam Books, 1984), pp. 26, 29, 102, 103.

53. Jane E. Brody, "Moderate Exercise . . .," *The New York Times* (June 10, 1986).

54. Rudolph Ballentine, M.D., *Diet and Nutrition* (Honedale, PA: The Himalayan International Institute, 1978), p. 170.

55. Philip M. Boffey, "Coffee Drinking," *The New York Times* (November 12, 1985), p. C1.

56. Associated Press "5-Cup Coffee Habit Tied to Lung Cancer," *San Francisco Chronicle* (June 24, 1985) p. 19.

57. "Groups Want Coffee-decaffeinator Banned," *USA Today* (June 9, 1986), p. 40.

58. Marian Burros, "A Sweetener's Effects," *The New York Times* (July 3, 1985), p. C1.

59. *Harvard Medical School Health Letter*, (January 1986).

60. "Alcohol . . .," *The Journal of the American Medical Association*, vol. 225, no. 17 (May 2, 1986), p. 2311.

61. Philip Collins, "Water: Do You Drink Enough?" *The Mother Earth News*, (September/October 1983).

62. "Beware Water Diets," *The New York Times* (February 17, 1985), p. C2.

63. Oliver Alabaster, M.D., Op. cit., p. 50.

64. Steven F. Maier and Mark Laudenslager, "Stress and Health: Exploring the Links," *Psychology Today*, (August 1985), p. 44.

65. "Healthy Feet," pamphlet published by Kinney Shoes.

66. ———, "House Plants Filter Out Air Pollution, Says Researcher," *The New York Times* (September 3, 1985) p. C3.

67. David Margolick, "Anti-smoking Climate Inspires Suits by the Dying," *The New York Times* (March 15, 1985).

68. "Cancer in Passive Smokers," *The New York Times* (July 9, 1985).

69. Lindsey Gruson, "Employers Get Tough on Smoking At Work," *The New York Times* (March 14, 1985), p. B1.

70. "Clearing the Air," National Cancer Institute Publication No. 84-1647. Available from National Cancer Institute, Bethesda MD 20205.

71. Susan Gilbert, "Noise Pollution," *Science Digest*, (March 1985) p. 28.

72. Sheldon Cohen, "Sound Effects Behavior," *Psychology Today*, (October 1981), pp. 38-43.

73. Steven Halpern with Louis Savory, *Sound Health: The Music and Sounds That Make Us Whole* (San Francisco: Harper and Row, 1985), p. 125.

74. David M. Lipscomb, *The Healing Energies of Music* (Wheaton, Illinois: Theosophical Publishing House, 1983).

75. Hal Hellman, "Guiding Light," *Psychology Today*, (April 1982), p. 27.

76. "Reports from Research," Duro-Test Corporation, Form 968 (1984).

77. "Time Troubles," *The Medical Forum*, Harvard Medical School Health Letter, vol. VII, no. 9 (July 1982), p. 3.

78. Jane E. Brody, "Surprising Health Impact Discovered for Light," *The New York Times* (December 13, 1984), p. C1.

79. Ibid.

80. "Light and Health," Duro-Test Corporation press release (May 1985).

81. Hal Hellman, "Guiding Light," *Psychology Today* (April 1982), pp. 22-28.

82. Jeff Meer, "The Light Touch," *Psychology Today*, (September 1985), p. 63.

83. Carole Jackson, *Color Me Beautiful* (New York: Ballantine Books, 1980).

84. Garrison Keillor, "Prairie Home Companion," National Public Radio (November 16, 1985).

85. Daniel Goleman, "Analyst Creates Therapy," *The New York Times* (July 2, 1985), p. C1.

86. Linda Hoeschler, interview with author, Minneapolis, MN, February, 1985.

87. David Dovenberg, interview with author, Minneapolis, MN, February, 1985.

88. Daniel Goleman, "Relaxation: Surprising Benefits Detected," *The New York Times* (May 13, 1986).

89. Steven F. Maier and Mark Laudenslager, "Stress and Health: Exploring the Links," *Psychology Today*, (August 1985), p. 49.

90. *Today's Health*, (David McClelland and colleagues) (July/August 1985), p. 19.

91. Daniel Goleman, "Concentration Is Likened to Euphoric States of Mind," *The New York Times* (March 4, 1986), p. C1.

92. "WordSpinning" is a title of my own invention for a technique I've been using for years as a "round outline" in preparation for dramatic writing. A similar technique, which he calls "The Lotus Meditation," is used by the Rev. Robert Corin Morris when working with groups. Tony Buzan described his similar process as "mapping" in his 1976 book *Use Both Sides of the Brain.* Dr. Gabriele Lusser Rico calls her method "clustering" in her book *Writing the Natural Way* (Los Angeles: J. P. Tarcher, 1983).

93. John Boyle, lecture, *The Omega Seminar*, (The Institute for Executive Research, 1974).

94. Wording of some affirmations suggested by Erik Esselstyn, Ed.D., Micki Esselstyn, M.S.W., Joie Bourisseau and Rhoda Semel.

95. Penny Jacobs, interview with author, Minneapolis, MN, February 1985.

96. Bernie Seigel, M.D., lecture "The Art of Healing", The Association for Humanist Psychology, Philadelphia, (May 1985).

97. O. C. and S. Simonton, *Getting Well Again* (Los Angeles: J. P. Tarcher, 1982).

98. Steven F. Maier and Mark Laudenslager, "Stress and Health: Exploring the Links," *Psychology Today*, (August 1985), p. 49.

99. Mary Jasnoski, a pychologist, reported these findings at a 1986 meeting of the Society of Behavioral Medicine in San Francisco.

100. Joseph Chilton Pearce, *The Bond of Power* (New York: Elsevier-Dutton) *Brain/Mind Bulletin*, (July 13, 1981).

101. E. J. Dionne, Jr., "Pope Meets Dalai Lama," *The New York Times*, February 3, 1986.

102. Pandit Usharbudh Arya, D. Litt., lecture "Meditation", The Himalyan Institute, Honesdale, PA, March, 1982.

103. Interweave Center, *Meditation Handbook #1*, Interweave Center, 422 Clark Street, South Orange, NJ 07079.

104. Some of the ideas on meditation variation in this section are derived from conversations with the Rev. Robert Corin Morris.

105. Some of the ideas on expressing anger in this section resulted from conversations with mental health consultant Dr. Donna Gaffney.

106. George Krebs, Ph.D., Interweave stress management workshop, May 3, 1985.

107. Martin Luther King, Jr., *Strength to Love* (Fortress Press, 1963).

108. Val Prescott, interview with author, Minneapolis MN, February 25, 1985.

109. These ideas for expressing anger were generated in a workshop conducted by Erik Esselstyn, Ed. D., and Micki Esselstyn, M.S.W., for Interweave Center.

110. Many of the ideas in this chapter were discussed at Interweave Center workshops. Erik Esselstyn, Ed.D., Micki Esselstyn, M.S.W., Barbara Krebs, Ph.D., George Krebs, Ph.D., and Robert Corin Morris, M.Div., were group leaders.

111. Cathy M. West, Ph.D., provided the "rules for arguing."

112. John Liebeskind, Yehuda Shavit, et al., "Endorphins Connected with Stress-related Cancer," *Brain/Mind Bulletin*, vol. 9, no. 9 (July 1984), p. 1.

113. Steven F. Maier and Mark Laudenslager, "Stress and Health: Exploring the Links," *Psychology Today*, (August 1985), p. 44.

114. Daniel Goleman, "Strong Emotional Response to Disease May Bolster Patient's Immune System," *The New York Times* (October 22, 1985), p. C1.

115. ——— "Brain Has Key Role in Heart Attacks," *Brain/Mind Bulletin*, vol. 9, no. 9 (July 1984) p. 3.

116. Jeffrey Mervis, "The Psychological Route to Cutting Costs," *The New York Times* (November 24, 1985).

117. Material in this section was derived from conversations with therapist Loretta Lewis, M.A., M.S., November 1985.

118. ———, "Job Autonomy . . .," *The New York Times*, (May 28, 1985), p. C1.

119. Paul Clancy, *USA Today*, (June 26, 1986) p. 1.

120. William Meyers, "Child Care Finds a Champion in the Corporation," *The New York Times* (August 4, 1985), p. 1.

121. Nadine Brozan, "Infant-care Leaves: Panel Urges Policy," *The New York Times* (November 28, 1985).

122. ———, "18-Week Leave for New Parents Urged in Congress," *The New York Times* (March 6, 1986), p. C7.

123. Benton & Bowles, Inc., "Men's Changing Role," *American Consensus*; reported in *Leading Edge*, vol. 8, (Jaunuary 12, 1981).

124. Maxi-listmaking idea from therapist Kathy Win. M.S.W., clinical therapist at Raritan Bay Mental Health Center, Perth Amboy, N.J.

298

125. Daniel Goleman, "Clues to Suicide: A Brain Chemical Is Implicated," *The New York Times* (October 8, 1985), p. C1.

126. ——— "The Optimal Coffee Break," *Psychology Today*, (April 1985), p. 21.

127. Alan Beck and Aaron Katcher, "Four-legged Therapists," *Discover*, (August 1983), p. 88.

128. Lois Rosenthal, "The Birmingham Will," *Writers Digest*, (June 1985), p. 28.

129. John Boyle, The Omega Seminar, "Self-Esteem," Telemark Lodge, Cable, WI., 1975.

130. Jeffrey Zaslow, "Fourth-grade Girls These Days Ponder Weighty Matters," *The Wall Street Journal* (Feb 1, 1986), p. 1.

131. Daniel Goleman, "Dislike of Own Body Found Common Among Women," *The New York Times* (March 19, 1985), p. C1.

132. April Fallon, Ph.D., and Paul Rozin, Ph.D., *Journal of Abnormal Psychology*, (March 1985).

133. ———, "The Trouble with Dieting," *American Health*, (Jan/Feb 1985).

134. Gloria Arenson, *Binge Eating* (New York: Rawson Associates, 1984).

135. William Bennett, M.D. and Joel Gurin, *The Dieter's Dilemma,* (New York: Basic Books, 1982).

136. John Morley, "Endorphins Key to Obesity, Peak in Pregnancy," *Psychoneuroendocrinology* (361-379); reported in *Brain/Mind Bulletin*, (May 7, 1984), p. 3.

137. Many of the ideas on appetite satisfaction in this section were developed in conversations with therapist Loretta Lewis, M.A., M.S.

138. Sheila Fields, *Bulimia: A Common Problem at University of Wisconsin* (doctoral thesis); reported by Diane Zelman in the *Ada James Women's Center Newsletter*, vol. 010, no. 030 (Autumn 1985), p. 11.

139. American Anorexia/Bulimia Association, Inc. newsletter, (June-August 1984).

140. Cathy M. West, Ph.D., provided this information.

141. Gloria Arenson, *Binge Eating*, (New York: Rawson Associates, 1984).

142. Adapted from Alan Lakein's *How to Get Control of Your Time and Your Life*, (New York: N.A.L., 1974).

143. Martha Burgess, interview with author, Bethesda, MD, October 1985.

144. EST, now called The Forum, is a transformational workshop.

145. DMA is a workshop on the creative process.

146. Loretta Lewis, M.A., M.S., interview with author, New Jersey, December 1985.

147. Rabindranath Tagore quote, *Spiritual Diary* (Honesdale, PA: Himalayan Publishers).

148. Lisa Berkman and S. Leonard Syme, "Social Networks, Host Resistance, and Mortality: A Nine-year Follow-up of Alameda County Residents, "*The American Journal of Epidemiology*, (1979 109:20), pp. 186-204.

149. K. B. Nuckolls, J. Cassel, and B. H. Kaplan, "Psychosocial Assets, Life Crisis, and the Prognosis of Pregnancy," *The American Journal of Epidemiology*, vol. 95, (1972), pp. 431-41.

150. The Rev. Robert Corin Morris, executive director, Interweave Center, Summit NJ 07901, interview with author, May 1985.

151. Joie Bourisseau, energy management consultant, interview with author, Washington, D.C., October 30, 1985.

152. Janice Howard, interview with author, San Diego, CA, June 1985.

153. "Let There Be Peace on Earth," an interview with Jill Jackson Miller, *Science of Mind Today*, vol. 2, no. 2, (Winter 1985), p. 5.

154. Jessica Lipnack and Jeffrey Stamps, *Networking* (Garden City: Doubleday and Company, Inc., 1982). Reprinted in *Holistic Living* (August/September 1983) p. 9.

155. Pierre Teihard de Chardin, *Human Energy* (London: William Collins Sons & Co. Ltd., 1969), p. 154.

156. Ken Keyes, Jr., *The One Hundredth Monkey* (Coos Bay, Oregon: Vision Books).

157. ———, "Grass Roots Movement Seeks to Change People's Thinking About War . . .," *PR Reporter*, vol. 28, no. 10 (March 11, 1985), p. 1.

Phyllis Paullette, who holds an advanced degree from Columbia University, has been an active advocate for purer and more nutritious foods, a yoga teacher, an award-winning filmmaker and an adjunct college professor. An associate of Interweave Center in Summit, N.J., she leads workshops in Energistics and writes on a variety of subjects.

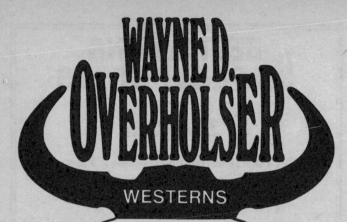

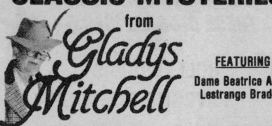

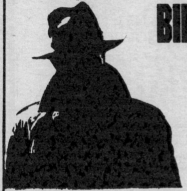